Man Cannot Live on
Vitamins Alone

Man Cannot Live on Vitamins Alone

—how vitamin supplements & corporate politics adversely affect your health

Dr. Vic Shayne

Writers Club Press

San Jose   New York   Lincoln   Shanghai

Man Cannot Live on Vitamins Alone
—how vitamin supplements & corporate
politics adversely affect your health

Writers Club Press
an imprint of iUniverse, Inc.

For information address:
iUniverse, Inc.
5220 S. 16th St., Suite 200
Lincoln, NE 68512
www.iuniverse.com

ISBN: 0-595-23654-5

Printed in the United States of America

CONTENTS

ACKNOWLEDGMENTS

In every book I read there is a page full of acknowledgments. I used to open to the page, read a few sentences then move on. The friends and family of the author are relatively meaningless to anyone other than a close circle of people. So here is your out. If you don't know me, skip ahead to the first page of the important stuff and get into the meat of things. But if you've helped me along the way with this project, take a moment to relish the thought that I am sending out to you.

First I am thanking my wife, Janice, who frequently commented to me, "What? You're writing another book? Come away from that computer already!" Next, thanks to my children, Josh and Tasha, who used to be little children, but now are almost as old as I am. This book should show them that if you are stubborn and obsessed, you can write a bunch of books, which must be good for something. Thanks, Tasha, for keeping those emails coming from Project Censored; it's good to know that someone's keeping an eye on environmental polluters and politicians speaking out of both sides of their lobbyists' mouths. And thanks, Josh, for always being there to help me with my computer problems, including the time you valiantly tried to knock me unconscious with a wheel of aged blue cheese to keep me from throwing my computer into a nearby canal.

Special thanks goes also to my friend Judy Goodman who did as she promised, reading this book for grammatical errors. Not only have you kept your word, but you were brutal in your comments, which were greatly appreciated. One of the things which you did for me was to eradicate the word "which," which I used too much. As a retired English teacher, you shamelessly forced me to further explain myself and add substantiation for my claims in a number of instances, adding to both my credibility and the addition of extra words, commas and dashes, for whatever good that did. If there are any errors whatsoever (if I may use this word), I hold you harmless and am willing to sign a contract to that effect. Does anyone know a good lawyer? Regardless, I hope this project has given you some *upliftment.* (This word can be found only in a very large dictionary).

Lastly, I thank my brother Gordon who thought so much of my last book that he used it under his patio table to keep it from wobbling. This should prove to the world that my books really are practical.

Well, this is about as lighthearted as this book gets. Now for the heavy stuff…

"*Unlike the Greek-trained Western mind, the Chinese mind does not aim at grasping details for their own sake, but at a view which sees the detail as part of a whole.*

This grasping of the whole is obviously the aim of science as well, but it is a goal that necessarily lies very far off because science, whenever possible, proceeds experimentally and in all cases statistically. Experiment, however, consists in asking a definite question which excludes as far as possible anything disturbing and irrelevant. It makes conditions, imposes them on Nature, and in this way forces her to give an answer to a question devised by man. She is prevented from answering out of the fullness of her possibilities since these possibilities are restricted as far as practicable. For this purpose there is created in the laboratory a situation which is artificially restricted to the question and which compels Nature to give an unequivocal answer. The workings of Nature in her unrestricted wholeness are completely excluded. If we want to know what these workings are, we need a method of inquiry which imposes the fewest possible conditions, or if possible no conditions at all and then leaves Nature to answer out of her fullness."[1]

—Dr. Carl Jung

[1] Jung, Carl, *Synchronicity*, Bollingen Foundation, NY 1960

NATURAL & SCIENTIFIC CREATIONS CAN NEVER BE THE SAME

What's the difference between something natural and something human-made? Nature is based on an intricate, living, interdependent, interrelated system—a variety and synergy too vast, complex and dynamic to ever be duplicated by scientists. Variety is not only the spice of life, it is also its strength and the nature of its spirit and mystery. Attempted improvements to Nature's design always create side effects and imbalances because human beings cannot perceive the complexity and variables that are disturbed through their interference; nor can human beings foresee the long and short term effects caused by scientific intervention, tweaking, tampering and experimentation. Fooling with the design and flow of Mother Nature is guaranteed to stir her wrath, to use a mythological model. When a scientist tells us that human-made vitamins are the same as those found in Nature's foods, then that scientist is drowning in his/her own sea of arrogance and lack of insight.

Few of us have problems perceiving the difference between a living tree in the woods and a fake plant decorating a corner of a room; or between a juicy orange and an orange-flavored candy. We innately know why natural things are health-promoting while human-made creations are questionable in their design. When we ingest a food we are taking into our bodies the wonders and mysteries of Nature. Real foods are comprised of a *complex* array of nutrients, flavors, aromas and nurturing energy that scientists can never duplicate, because the secrets of the universe—so vast, complicated

1

and interwoven—are bound up in the living energy of every natural food. This is why they nurture our bodies like no other substances. We can trust in Nature, while we always must question the end-products produced in laboratories.

Most modern peoples, growing up far from the world of farms, food cultivation, seed planting and the great outdoors, rarely stop to ponder the awesome role of Nature's foods in our health and healing. The healing power of Nature is rarely appreciated in our modern world. We are thoroughly inundated with marketing messages, drug usage and our current form of health care usually mandating that the patient surrenders his/her treatment to the doctor without taking a proactive role *after* sickness has already set in. Patients look to doctors to "fix" them, yet rarely work to build their own health *before* they are ill and suffering. This is a backwards approach to health care. In the ideal scenario, we should understand the properties of nature's foods and learn how to keep ourselves healthy by consuming them. We have bodies, but we don't have a clue as to how they work and how to maintain them properly. Of course, we have learned that, by going to work-out at the gym, we can keep weight off, tone our muscles and improve our respiratory and cardiovascular systems. We also know that if we bathe frequently we can keep our skin clean and healthy. If we brush our teeth, maybe we can prevent bad breath and a few cavities. But these are all superficial facets of health. By looking closer, we must pay attention to deeper concerns, often unseen and hidden deep within our tissues, organs and musculoskeletal systems. We need to commit to a serious and lasting relationship that fosters a strong connection between all of our bodies' systems and the foods we eat.

Foods Contain A "Complex" of Many Nutrients

Lendon Smith, M.D., one of America's most outspoken physicians of the baby boomer era, explains:

All the research has found that we animals are bags of water with vitamins, minerals, enzymes, hormones, proteins, fats and sugar floating about therein. Over the centuries of experimenting, humans have found which of nature's flora (and some fauna) do *what*. Now with sophisticated biochemical analysis we are able to understand the *why*. Tests can determine what vitamins and minerals and oils are in the plants and in what proportions. Sure, we know about carrots and vitamin A and night blindness. Yes, we know about the calming effect of calcium and magnesium-bearing foods. Okay, so magnesium will help insomnia (magnesium is necessary to build chlorophyll, the green in plants), and relieve jumpiness, control muscle cramps, reduce craving for chocolate and raise one's threshold to noise. When an herb has been found to do these things, then we know it at least has magnesium in it. But just taking magnesium may not be enough. **It is as if nature knew what other elements were necessary to be incorporated in the plant to make it tastier or more absorbable.** There are reasons for everything.[2]

Dr. Smith tells us "there are reasons for everything," yet we choose to ignore the reasons Nature's foods are comprised of a "complex" of nutrients. Food contains nutrients that we cannot get in any other way, not even through vitamin and mineral supplements! We should all know and understand this so we can prevent illness, promote good health, protect our bodies from environmental and chemical assault, and support our cells. Such knowledge would be empowering, enabling us to control and direct the destiny of our personal health—taking an active role in feeding our cells the nutrients they demand for optimal health. Nutrients are found in the foods produced in Nature. Exactly how and why they work is

---

[2] Heinerman, John, *Heinerman's Encyclopedia of Fruits, Vegetables & Herbs*, Parker Publishing, NY 1988, page x

still mostly a mystery, but this does not invalidate their importance and efficacy. We cannot explain how the sun came into existence and continues to radiate us with its energy, but this doesn't mean that we do not need the sun or that the sun doesn't have the power to give life to our planet and all its inhabitants. Nature is poorly understood; it does not tolerate artificial manipulation, and works at its own pace. These facts tend to frustrate impatient people (the majority of us living in these modern times) who want quick results, high potency and on-demand action.

It's just too bad that we have been driven so off course by our scientific and medical "advances" that we as a modern society fail to recognize the immense importance and healing power of Nature's nutrient-dense foods. Instead, we have usurped Nature by relying on immature, unpredictable, side-effect-causing, unbalanced chemicals and surgical responses to health problems. We have, as a society, abandoned health care in favor of medical care. With our live-for-today attitude, we choose to ignore that tomorrow is sure to arrive and catch us unprepared and unaware. We cannot forget that our bodies are natural entities and respond best to natural health solutions. We are not robots who can thrive on synthetic oils, parts of foods, extracts and replacement parts. Financially lucrative and convenient solutions at best keep us going like temporary patches on old bicycle tires, never really addressing the underlying causes of our problems. We must have nutrients from Nature's food bounty to live, thrive and heal. This is a statement of natural law, not philosophy or radical thought. Food heals, energizes, nurtures and protects us against illness, pain, premature aging, degeneration and suffering (not only of the body, but of the mind and emotions as well).

Where the Notion Comes From

Where did the idea come from—that foods contain nutrients to heal and nurture the human body? If we look back into history, the answer is that our hairy ancestors discovered that certain plants, herbs and roots cured sickness and injury. In our modern era, food science researchers have confirmed the healing and prevention power of our plant kingdom. This is a common denominator of so-called "modern" medical health care and so-called "natural" health care. The highly esteemed medical text *Merck Manual* (published every year since 1898) tells us that vitamins, minerals and other nutrients come from foods and are essential to our health. No mention is made of any vitamin without citing the natural foods wherein they are found. For example, under the heading "Vitamin A," *Merck Manual* states:

> Vitamin A (retinol) is fat soluble and is found mainly in fish liver oils, liver, egg yolk, butter and cream. Green leafy and yellow vegetables contain b-carotene and other provitamin carotenoids that undergo central fission of the molecule in the mucosal cells of the small intestine to form retinol...[3]

This textbook does not say that vitamin A is found in pills, but rather foods.

Further, *Merck Manual* states:

> The importance of nutrition in clinical medicine is increasingly acknowledged, partly due to the recognition that malnutrition frequently occurs in prolonged illness and may accompany acute injury and complicated surgical and medical procedures. Many genetic metabolic disorders require special diets for their management. There is also an increased understanding of the role of nutritional factors in degenerative disorders. Deficiency states such as marasmus, kwashiorkor and xerophthalmia continue to form a major part of clinical practice in developing countries,

---

[3]. *Merck Manual of Diagnosis and Therapy*, 16th Edition, Merck Research Laboratories, NJ, 1992, p. 959

but these and other deficiencies may occur anywhere under conditions of deprivation.[4]

There we have it—one of the most respected books in all of modern medicine refers to foods as having healing and illnesss-prevention power. One has to wonder if modern-day doctors and other health practitioners actually read and study their own text books, or whether they choose to ignore nutritionally-based science because it is not as lucrative or exclusive as using drugs and surgeries to address health problems. Or maybe they are like the rest of us in society who grow up listening to studies and news reports touting the marvels of wonder drugs and medical "advances" to the point where we are misled to believe that such practices are better than nature's foods for addressing our health needs. And why do we ignore the reality that such pseudo-solutions *never* prevent illness from occurring in the first place?

We erroneously have been led to believe that man, through scientific invention, is capable of outdoing nature and understanding the infinite and dynamic complexity of nature and nature's foods. We are even misled to believe that a vitamin can be "natural" when it is no longer still contained in its original food form! The word "natural" has been bastardized, no longer resembling its original meaning of being a part of Nature. It has all but lost its clear, pure, pristine, complex meaning. That which has been extracted, isolated, added to, fortified and chemicalized at the hands of scientists is not natural. Hence, **any vitamin that is no longer contained in its original food cannot be truly natural**.

There is no doubt that we have been so inundated with marketing messages—advertisements and magazine and news articles—that we question that which is natural while readily accepting man-made chemicals as health-promoting. It is due to marketing that the mere thought that food can cure illness and prevent disease is ludicrous to most Americans and far

---

[4.] ibid, pages 940–941

too many doctors. As a nation of drugs, fast foods and medical-dependency, we are ignorant of the healing power of Nature to the point where even our learned experts—doctors and scientists—tell us without hesitation and with great confidence that foods cannot cure our ills. I have been told this by several health care practitioners who are supposed to know enough to help me and my family. Ignorance is a dangerous thing, especially when it is in the possession of our health care providers.

We're Talking About Nutrition, Naturally

This book is about nutrition, health and healing, and the complexity and interrelationships of nature and the individual. Mostly, however, this is an exploration of the wonders of nutrition. Before we go any further, let me qualify what I mean by the word "nutrition" by saying that what some people consider to be the practice of nutrition is what I would consider the practice of pharmacology (the use of drug-like chemicals in treating disease and symptoms). In the strictest sense, nutrition implies the consumption (eating) of nature's real, whole, natural foods to glean a wide array of nutrients to be used by our bodies for many purposes and functions. Nutrition is about feeding our cells the raw materials they need to work effectively and efficiently, which in turn keeps us healthy. Nutrition comes from Nature's foods. But this is NOT how most practitioners in the field of nutrition act, practice or preach. To the contrary, most people, including practitioners, think of vitamins, minerals and other supplements BEFORE they think of foods when you mention the subject of nutrition. Chances are that people may never even think about food when they ponder the word nutrition; they may just think of vitamins. The concept of nutrition has shifted from Nature's foods in favor of human-made chemicals that are little different from drugs, even if we call these chemicals "natural" vitamins.

When people visit my office complaining of any one of thousands of health problems, I first entertain the most natural solutions possible. I immediately begin to consider the roles of the foods and nonfoods in their daily diet, stress, environmental toxins, air and water quality in their lives and their mental and emotional states. To the contrary, however, I have noticed that most practitioners (nutritionists, doctors, nurses, dietitians, physicians, etc.) gravitate toward chemical answers to health questions. They begin to formulate a protocol incorporating very specific drugs, vitamins, minerals, amino acids, coenzymes, enzymes, antioxidants and bioflavonoids. These non-food, unnatural solutions arise because the very concept of nutrition is now associated with chemicals, of which vitamins lead the field. But vitamins are only small parts of nutrition; vitamins exist within foods, never in isolation (by themselves) in nature. Chemicals are scientific creations that should never be confused with or associated with the practice of nutrition. Even if a vitamin has been extracted out of a natural food, it is no longer really natural. Once it has been removed from its original food, in its naturally balanced and harmonious form, it can no longer share specific relationships and synergistic tasks with other nutrients and cofactors.

In this book we focus on real, natural nutrition involving vitamins, minerals and other food factors still found within Nature's foods. We'll explore how food nutrients differ from isolated chemicals (vitamins, minerals, et. al.) and how these two entities—food nutrients and chemicals—should never be confused or used carelessly as if they are the same thing. They are not. Nutrition is about the nutrients within foods, not about chemicals in pills.

There are many other nutritionists and doctors who agree with the concept that nutrients should be consumed as they exist within natural foods. Like me, they are adamant about the fact that there are ingredients within foods that are as important as vitamins for our health and healing. These nutritional ingredients are all but ignored by scientists and those practitioners seeking health solutions from chemically isolated vitamins and other substances that are no longer part of the food or have been created in a laboratory. Here are some comments by food nutrient advocates who convey the differences between chemicals and food nutrients:

"Natural vitamins are those occurring in food…Nutritionists often recommend obtaining vitamins from foods for several reasons…Foods supply mixtures of vitamins, minerals and other materials that may have beneficial effects. Mixtures are what the body uses. Foods supply materials that are not vitamins, yet are important. In this class are flavonoids, which work together with vitamin C to build strong capillaries and serve as antioxidants and as anti-inflammatory agents."[5]

A nutrient is a "food that supplies the body with its necessary elements."[6]

Vitamins are "biological complexes, bundles of enzymes and trace minerals, biological wheels within wheels within wheels. Trying to identify a vitamin in terms of a single chemical structure is self-defeating, because you have to have the whole complex to get the vitamin to function. The failure of the pharmaceutical approach to vitamins originated in the chemists' synthetic isolation of a single element uncombined with its biological matrix. But the discovery of the vitamins coincided with the boom in industrial, agricultural and pharmaceutical chemistry, which was crowding its way into all facets of life But it was in the attempted duplication of living things, like artificial fertilizers or vitamins, that chemistry had it s most distorting influence."[7]

Annemarie Colbin, founder of New York's renowned Natural Gourmet Cookery School for Food and Health, writes:

---

[5] Ronzio, Ph.D., Robert, *The Encyclopedia of Nutrition & Good Health*, Facts on File, NY 1997, p. 442

[6] Taber, Clarence wilbur, *Taber's Cyclopedic Medical Dictionary*, 9th Edition, F.A. Davis Co. Philadelphia, page N-34

[7] Bernard Jensen & Mark Anderson, *Empty Harvest*, Avery Publishing, NY, 1995, p. 125

Nature—our nature—abhors an imbalance…Fragmentation affects foods not only on the cellular, but also on the chemical level. When wheat is refined into white flour, for example, not only does it lose its bran and germ, but some twenty nutrients are also lost or greatly reduced. Enriching the flour—which entails returning four of those twenty nutrients—does not solve the problem. Not only are the added nutrients fewer in number than those present in the original whole wheat; they also lack the **energy** [emphasis added] they had when they were simply part of a living, growing plant. It's like cutting off your arm and then fitting you with a prosthetic one—it may have the same form and fulfill some of the same functions, but it is hardly as good as the original. Isolating the components of a living organism and then remixing them will not recreate the living organism.

The logic, to me, seems obvious: *Added nutrients do not contribute to a live energy field.*

In the ecosystem, the living creatures that comprise it are designed to subsist by consuming what the environment provides…Whole foods are simply fresh, natural, edible things, as close to their natural state as possible.[8]

Plant researcher/author James Duke, Ph.D. tells us that plant food and herbs provide nutrients that "are essential to life. Research has now shown that many of us are deficient in several nutrients essential to optimal health, if not essential to life itself. Many of these important, natural ingredients are found in herbs, but not in synthetic pharmaceuticals. Dr. Duke writes,"When synthetic drugs are made from plants, we tend to isolate one or another chemical and throw away the rest of the plant and its

---

8. Colbin, Annemarie, *Food & Healing*, Ballentine Books, NY, 1996, pages 36–38.

medicinal potential. The fava bean, for instance, contains ingredients that could be extracted and used as 'magic-bullet' pharmaceuticals—such as L-dopa, which is used in the treatment of Parkinson's Disease…But why throw away the rest of the bean to make a proprietary monochemical medicine that can be patented by a pharmaceutical company? We should, instead, be studying the synergistic energies of all those phytochemicals and discovering how they work so well together. Those are the studies that will lead us to a true understanding of the many healing qualities of medicinal plants."[9]

In essence, then, we must take a new, refreshing look at the concept of nutrition. It is time to reestablish the link between nutrition and food by considering that whole, raw, natural food alone contains live, complete and complex ingredients that are just not to be found in vitamin pills. Without these interactive, interrelated ingredients, there is no real nutrition, only pharmacology—aiming chemicals at diseases and symptoms. Our goal in the field of nutrition is to nutrify, or feed, the body as natural foods alone have the capacity to do.

[9.] Duke, Ph.D., James, *The Green Pharmacy*, Rodale Press, Pennsylvania, 1997.

COMING TO TERMS WITH NATURAL HEALTH CARE

Most every field of specialty has its own jargon. Following are some important words and phrases to help you understand the author's concepts. These terms are used frequently and possibly may be unfamiliar to the reader in the context of our discussion. This book is purposefully written to be nontechnical, yet it may occasionally be necessary to consult a dictionary or medical dictionary for further definition of words or phrases not mentioned, or perhaps not fully explained, in this section. Some terms not listed are defined in subsequent chapters as they are introduced.

Amino acids. The building blocks of proteins (in other words, proteins are made from amino acids which are substances found in protein-containing foods such as seeds, nuts, beans, raw milk and meats). There are many different amino acids that combine to create a protein; some of these must be present in the diet because we cannot produce them inside our bodies, and are therefore called essential amino acids.

Antioxidants. The substances in foods (certain vitamins, minerals, flavonoids, carotenoids, etc.) that keep cells from being damaged by oxygen-robbing molecules such as drugs, chemicals and pollutants.

Biochemistry. The field of biochemistry is a scientific approach to studying the behavior of living chemicals, molecules and other elements. The body's biochemistry refers to the body's mechanism (at the molecule level) of using food substances for nourishment and cellular function. Each natural food we eat contains a wide variety of nutrients which are then used by our body's cells for different functions, as our body breaks down nutrients into smaller parts (molecules) so they can be used and distributed throughout our systems.

Bioindividuality. The uniqueness of each individual with respect to all of the various aspects of a person's biological, physical, mental, emotional and spiritual make-up. Bioindividuality explains why "what's good for the goose" is not necessarily good for the gander. It explains why drugs, foods and vitamins have differing effects on each individual and these effects are not necessarily predictable or safe. Life is too complex and dynamic—always changing and evolving—for health care problems to be addressed with simple, singular and isolated chemicals that fail to incorporate the peculiarities and individualism that define and direct our entire health picture. The determination of how a substance (a drug, food or supplement) is to be used should also incorporate wisdom, experience, expertise and common sense.

Foul nutrition. Most of us have heard of *malnutrition* (lacking in adequate and proper nutrition to stay healthy), but few have seen the term *foul nutrition*, which describes the consumption of (non)foods that are bad for our health. Such foods are not **natural** foods and include chemicals, artificial sweeteners, pesticides, synthetic fertilizers, refined sugars, refined flours, food dyes, artificial flavors, emulsifiers, altered fats, hydrogenated and/or partially hydrogenated oils, artificial separators, chemical texturizers, and more. In many cases in the modern world, most of an individual's diet may be comprised of nonfoods—an entire diet made up of cooked, processed, altered and "dead" foods that are not natural by the time they are consumed. Foul nutrition leads to disease because our bodies are not equipped to deal with—and are greatly burdened by—chemical ingredients that have no nutritious benefit.

Glandulars. Many whole food supplements contain "glandulars," which are generally glands and organs of animals used as sources of nutrients. Although it was traditionally common for people to eat the glands and organs of animals up until very recently in the modern era [even in the United States], fewer and fewer people consume liver, kidney and other organs in their daily diets. But because glandulars contain important sources of nutrients (certain amino acids, whole proteins, minerals, vitamins, enzymes, etc.) that cannot be found in sufficient quantities in vegetarian diets, they are included in many whole food supplements to promote health, healing and immunity. To illustrate the nutritional value of glandulars, if we consider liver as a food, we see that it contains all of the following: Protein, Calcium, Iron, Magnesium, Phosphorus, Potassium, Zinc, Copper, Manganese, Selenium, Vitamin C complex, Vitamin B complex: Thiamin, Riboflavin, Niacin, Pantothenic acid, Folate, Vitamin B-12, Vitamin A, Vitamin D, Vitamin E; Lipids and Fatty acids; the Amino acids Tryptophan, Threonine, Isoleucine, Leucine, Lysine, Methionine, Cystine, Phenylalanine, Tyrosine, Valine, Arginine, Histidine, Alanine, Aspartic acid, Glutamic acid, Glycine, Proline and Serine. In addition there are other nutrients including enzymes, coenzymes (CoQ10), bioflavonoids, etc.[10]

Isolated vitamins. Real vitamins are found within (contained inside of) natural, whole foods. However, scientists have created a means of extracting vitamins out of natural foods and using them in therapies against symptoms. Isolated vitamins, therefore, are vitamins that no longer appear within their original foods; they are singular chemicals. Some isolated vitamins are synthetic—created in a laboratory to mimic the actions and structures of natural vitamins. Isolated vitamins, even if labeled "natural," are chemicals and not nutrients; they are not living nutrients and contain none of their natural synergists.

Marketing. Marketing refers to the way a product or service is sold, advertised and distributed to the public for consumption and/or use. All corporations and companies with a product or service must market them to be successful. As a result, marketing includes claims about products and services that are intended to motivate us as consumers to make purchases.

[10.] USDA Nutrient Database for Standard Reference, Release 13 (November 1999)

Sometimes the motivation is instilled by fear, such as the fear of NOT going to a medical doctor for a health problem or the fear of dying, or the fear of suffering or disfigurement. Fear is the primary emotion used to sell vaccinations, yearly check-ups, insurance policies, vitamins and drugs. Marketing messages and advertising are not necessarily truthful and are almost always slanted to be persuasive instead of informative. This is most confusing when the public is misled to believe that they are viewing a "news" report when, in actuality, they are watching or reading propaganda that is subtly promoting the use of drugs, medical treatment, vaccinations, or even the ever-elusive cure for cancer.

The term *marketing* may be applied in both negative and positive ways. Some products that are marketed to us certainly improve our lives, while others are harmful—or potentially harmful. Yet, despite a real or potential threat to our health, manufacturers work hard to get us to purchase their products, and will distort the truth, or outright lie, to separate us from our money. There are even many products that are both positive and negative, like automobiles that help us get around but also pollute the air and kill people on the highway. The difference between marketing "news" versus real news is objectivity and completeness of the presentation. For instance, an article on a new cure for cancer or AIDS would need to include all of the side effects from the treatment, as well as its unpredictability, its track record and the rest of its shortfalls. Equally important is the fair portrayal of how scientific research was conducted, and who sponsored the research. Marketing is the key to making products popular and to manipulating consumers into *believing* that such products are really good for us. Marketing and public relations professionals are "hired guns" to make their clients look good to the public, even if this means twisting the truth, omitting facts, presenting one-sided points-of-view, creating news, staging events or even slandering opponents. For an in-depth look at the way marketing and public relations firms work for their clients and influence public opinion, the reader is encouraged to study the book *Trust Us, We're Experts*, by Sheldon Rampton and John Stauber (prwatch.org).

Media. The media include newspapers, magazines, the Internet (websites), television networks and other avenues of communication. The major media in the United States are owned and operated by large corporations. Even though the media is privately owned, we as citizens too often rely on these sources for truthful information benefitting the public. Instead we are apt to receive marketing messages and biased corporate reporting. Understanding the role of the media in the free world is crucial when attempting to make wise decisions regarding your course of health care and the products and services you are influenced to buy. Today's media are dedicated to appeasing their advertisers, owners and business partners; and this is accomplished by publishing slanted (one-sided) news stories, defaming competitors, slandering scientists, and even financially backing specific political candidates who may further the cause of the corporations associated with the media. Most Americans severely underestimate the power and role of the media, because at one time the media in America boasted its right and determination to keep the public informed as a matter of exercising basic freedoms. A free society is an informed society, it has been traditionally argued. Now we must reevaluate the degree to which we are informed and *how*. As Americans, we have long relied on the media to be our ally; now we must see it for what it really is and question its agendas, partners and motivation. Media that fails to inform us of nuclear waste spills, the dangers of drugs, the risks of surgeries, tampering with the genetic codes of plant species and the availability of safer health care choices are not serving the public interest. This is what we are facing with today's modern media. We now must realize what the major television, radio and newspaper media really is—the voice of industry. And we must not be fooled into accepting information presented in these media as truthful, complete, healthful or even necessarily beneficial.

Natural. Natural is a term that has been misused for a long time. The most natural state is one wherein there has been no infringement by man's attempt to alter or improve any substance, food or plant. Companies marketing their products often will claim that they are natural even if their ingredients prove that MOST of their ingredients are synthetic chemicals while only a small percentage is made up of a natural compound. Natural health care, similarly, is not natural if it mixes herbs along with drugs. We cannot believe any manufacturer who states that a product is natural without doing our "homework" by carefully reading labels and questioning unfamiliar ingredients and their actions upon the human physiology and biochemistry. It may be difficult for many Americans to believe, but the truth is that many manufacturers lie to the consumer.

Nature. The word Nature throughout this book is written with a capital "N" unless quoted from another source. This is of purposeful design, meant to bring attention to the importance of Nature in this study. Spoken of with respect, Nature is not only a place, but perhaps more importantly, it is a concept—an idea—that reaches far beyond our conscious thought. Nature goes back into prehistoric times and is a state of being as much as a "thing." For some, the word Nature conjures up images of a pristine creek running through virgin woods; others may think of a white, sandy beach, a cloudless blue sky, birds in flight and the soothing sun. In terms of natural health care, Nature is meant to connote a standard of what is right and fitting for our bodies; it is the ideal state of being.

Nature nurtures with its innate intelligence and flow, taking the path of least resistance and utmost harmony and balance. Some may view Nature as an independent entity, having a "mind" of its own. Thus we may speak of the "innate intelligence" of Nature, referring to the seemingly brilliant way that Nature maintains balance, harmony, mystery and wonder in its ever-evolving, ever-unfolding process that shapes our lives on earth.

Nature is often referred to in the female gender. The concept of Nature as a nurturing mother figure goes back to ancient mythology with the recognition by early peoples of Nature's forces and ability to create and direct human life. In more modern times, even many scientists are embracing the Gaia principle, considering that the earth is actually a breathing entity and a macrocosm of all life forms on this planet. This is an interesting subject, but rests just beyond the focus of this book. In our study, Nature refers mostly to what is right and harmonious with our states of health in the most basic sense, relating to the correct foods we need for our bodies as well as the most peaceful, balanced and productive states of mind and emotions.

Nutrition. The practice of using natural, unaltered, complex foods to provide the body with substances required by cells to create biochemical balance and function to promote health, healing, immunity and prevention. By definition, a vitamin is only a nutrient when it still exists within its original food *complex*, not when it is isolated (pulled out of a food) and offered as a vitamin pill.

Pharmacology. Pharmacology is the science of using chemicals and chemical agents to achieve a change in physiology and thereby get rid of symptoms and disease. Drugs are pharmacological agents because they are not natural. Foods provide nutritional effects, while drugs and isolated vitamins provide pharmacological effects.

Physiology. The words **physiology** and **physiological function** denote how our bodies work mechanically, as opposed to chemically or biochemically. Physiology may refer to the function of a joint or the way our heart pumps blood throughout our bodies.

Synthetic vitamins. These are vitamins created in a laboratory, not in nature, to resemble natural vitamins. Synthetic vitamins are dead chemicals, not real nutrients and are not derived from foods.

Whole food. The term "whole food" is used to signify a natural food that is grown in nature and has not been appreciably altered by means of chemicals or heating or processing. Whole foods contain a host of important nutrients that we need for nourishing our cells and carrying on a wide range of functions that keep us healthy.

Whole food complex. Also termed **complex** or **food complex**, a whole food complex represents ALL of the ingredients that are found in a food, not just vitamins or minerals, but also fiber, pigments, chlorophyll, amino acids, enzymes and more. All of these parts of a food exist within a **complex**, because they exist in a way that they are dependent upon (and interwoven with) one another and are interrelated. For instance, although a vitamin is a part of the food complex, it does not exist alone, but rather in relation to other food substances that all work together, as a team, for a common purpose.

Whole Food Concentrate. A whole food concentrate supplement is a tablet, capsule or powder that is made by concentrating one or more whole foods into supplement form. Whole food concentrates represent a convenient, healthful way of ingesting a wide variety of important nutrients needed for many cellular, biochemical, physiological functions. They are not used to cure disease, but rather to support the body in its effort to overcome nutritional deficiencies associated with symptoms and disease.

THE NATURALIST-
WHOLIST PHILOSOPHY

In the beginning, to borrow a biblical phrase, human beings ate a natural diet. All of the foods they consumed were all-natural, completely without human-made chemicals, and were not even altered by cooking or processing. This was the most primitive, natural way of eating. Eating this way made human beings at one with their environment and other living creatures. Disease in those days was not the enemy it has now become, threatening life and lifestyles. Rather, the dreaded threat was from weather, fierce animals, competition for food and shelter, and accidents. Any disease that existed was primarily due to accidents and malnutrition—not getting enough of the right foods to eat.

Now, this picture of our world has turned upside-down. The biggest threat to life and health these days comes from the following main areas (NOT viral, bacterial or hereditary causes):

FOUL NUTRITION

It used to be malnutrition that led to our demise—or not enough of the right kinds of foods or even a short supply of food that led to famine. Today, however, foul nutrition is the mainstay, marked by the consumption of bad foods—foods that have been processed, stripped of their nutrients, altered through heating and chemical reactions, and injected with chemicals and/or containing chemical residues such as cancer-causing pesticides and synthetic fertilizers. "Foul nutrition" refers to a daily diet of foods that injure us and fail to provide us with the building blocks of health.

It has been argued that inadequate nutrition leads to a depressed immune system. This is a very important consideration, because the immune system—the mechanism by which our bodies protect themselves—is the way we defend ourselves against disease. Most diseases these days are blamed on theoretical causes such as viruses, bacteria, other germs and genetics. The studies pointing to these causes are incomplete, because they do not explain why some people get sick while others do not. If germs alone were the cause of disease, none of us would have survived to this point. Rather, the immune system is failing to protect us as designed by nature. But how can it protect us when we fill ourselves with chemicals, live in toxic environments and ingest nonfood diets?

TEMPERATURE EXTREMES

Exposure to temperature extremes also takes its toll on our health. What is often blamed on viruses causing cold and flu every winter and summer is actually sickness caused by exposure to extreme temperature changes. Our grandmothers and great grandmothers understood the idea of dressing warmly in the winter, or not "overheating" in the summer. Exposure to temperature changes shocks the body and can lead to illness. Just this past summer, the Minnesota Vikings professional football team lost a virile, young player named Korey Stringer to heat stroke, demonstrating the powerful effects of exposure to extreme temperature on the human physiology of even a highly conditioned athlete. The body thrives on a constant, protected temperature. By exposure to extreme temperature, the body is forced to regulate an often overwhelming external influence; and the result is illness, or "dis-ease." Further, historians are all too familiar with traditional outbreaks of tuberculosis and other respiratory diseases in the depth of winter, demonstrating the ill effects of cold weather on an unprepared culture, especially when conditions are combined with unsanitary living conditions.

EXPOSURE TO CHEMICALS

Chemicals by the thousands pollute our internal and external environments. We as natural human beings are not meant to be assaulted by chemicals such as pesticides, synthetic fertilizers, drugs, isolated and synthetic vitamins, birth control pills and synthetic hormones, paint and varnish fumes, automobile exhaust, asbestos dust, mercury dental fillings, lead from industrial waste, radioactive waste, altered and hydrogenated oils, fried fats, synthetic clothing and building materials, and so much more. Chemicals permeate our lives, entering our bodies through our skin, the air we breathe, the water we drink and bathe in, and the foods we eat. Such chemicals cause skin lesions, respiratory illness, nervous system damage, reproductive problems and hormonal imbalances, brain damage, joint problems, emotional disturbances, cardiovascular illness, and diseases ranging from cold and flu to cancer. There are so many chemicals in our food and environment that they are overwhelming our health faster than we can cope with them. Within the past few decades, this fact has led to a whole new branch of health care to address "multiple chemical sensitivities," wherein doctors work to understand the myriad ways their patients are overwhelmed by chemicals in their environments and their daily diets.

The dangers of chemical exposure to children is perhaps the most alarming of all realities. This was brought into public awareness by investigative journalist Bill Moyers in his PBS broadcast on Kids & Chemicals, May, 2002. Moyers said:

> In my lifetime, more than 75,000 synthetic chemicals and metals have been put to use in America. Chemicals, that in many cases, make our lives easier and better. They kill insects and weeds, clean our clothes and carpets, unclog our drains, create produce and lawns, pretty as a picture. But most of these chemicals have never been tested for their toxic effects on children. And scientists are concerned that recent increases in childhood illnesses like asthma and cancer, as well as, learning disabilities,

may be related to the environment—to what kids eat, drink and breathe...Of the 3000 or so high production volume chemicals in use in this country today only 43% have been even minimally tested. Only about 10 percent have been thoroughly tested to examine their potential effects on children's health and development. So little testing has left scientists and policy makers in the dark about the toxicity of thousands of chemicals...

Dr. Philip Landrigan is a pioneer in the emerging field of children's environmental health. From New York's Mount Sinai School of Medicine he works with scientists around the country to understand how kids are affected by exposure to chemicals.

DR. LANDRIGAN: Fifty or 60 years ago in this country the major diseases in children were the infectious diseases...Today the major causes of illness in kids are chronic diseases...We know that chemicals in the environment are responsible for some of these effects. We know, for example, that some cases of development disability in children are caused by exposures to lead, to pesticides, to mercury, to PCBs. We suspect that children who are exposed to pesticides are at greater risk of childhood cancer than other children. But mostly we don't know.[11]

As long as corporations continue to produce life-threatening chemicals on purpose and/or as a byproduct of their industries, they will continue to poison us in countless ways. What's worse is the fact that many of these polluting industrial giants sponsor cancer and disease research that looks everywhere for the "cause" except right in the corporation's backyard. Instead of studying the effects of chemicals as cancer-causers, industry-sponsored cancer researchers are looking for viruses, vaccines and genetic links. The reason for this is rather obvious, if you consider the benefits of creating a smoke screen that keeps the attention of U.S. citizens focused

---

[11.] NOW with Bill Moyers, PBS transcript, May 10, 2002.

anywhere but on the producers of cancer-causing substances. Corporations producing toxic waste and carcinogenic products find it bad for business if Americans were to discover that cancer comes from their industry. By sponsoring "research" to "prove" or theorize that cancer is caused by genetics and viruses, they can continue to reap their huge profits without public outcry. Meanwhile, millions of Americans continue to suffer and die at the hands of corporate evil, the most un-American of all activities. To understand the complexity of this issue, how industry continues to poison our lives, and why scientists are looking in all the wrong places—or are paid to look in all the wrong places, consider this:

> Rather than efforts to identify environmental causes affecting cancer rates…much of the scientific research and public discussion has focused on treatments—the so-called 'race for the cure.' On paper, about a third of the U.S. National Cancer Institute's $2 billion annual budget is dedicated to prevention research, but those are 'rubber numbers,' according to longtime cancer researcher John C. Bailar III of MicGill University. Most of what the institute calls 'prevention' is actually basic research into the cellular mechanisms of cancer development rather than epidemiological studies and prevention trials. Research into cellular mechanisms and molecular biology has yet to accomplish much by way of saving lives, but it is politically safe research because it doesn't rock many boats. A researcher who studies cell biology doesn't have to risk getting hammered by the tobacco industry, agribusiness, or chemical manufacturers. 'The prevention of cancer on a big scale is going to require that we change our habits, change our life styles, clean up the work place, clean up the environment, change the consumer products that contain hazardous materials,' says Bailar.[12]

---

12. Rampton, Sheldon and John Stauber, *Trust Us, We're Experts!* Tarcher/Putnam Books, 2001, p. 145.

Without regard to human health and lifestyle, the world's largest chemical-producing companies are destroying neighborhoods, habitat, the environment and generations to come without conscience. One such example of this was recently reported in *The New York Times*, revealing that chemical giant Monsanto, for nearly 40 years has been dumping toxic polychlorinated biphenyls (PCBs) despite the known toxicity of these chemicals. Over the four decades, the *Times* reported:

> St. Louis-based Monsanto flushed tens of thousands of pounds of PCBs and other toxic wastes into Snow Creek [Anniston, Alabama] each year, sending the chemicals meandering through long-established neighborhoods and into Chccolocco Creek. More than 45 tons of PCBs, a highly efficient industrial insulator, were discharged in 1969 alone, according to company documents. Monsanto also deposited millions of pounds of PCBs in a hillside landfill just above the plant.

> Thirty miles away, in Gadsden, Ala., a jury is hearing a lawsuit filed by…more than 3,500…plantiffs who contend that Monsanto and its chemical division, Solutia Inc., should compensate them for reduced property values, emotional distress and, in some cases, health problems related to the PCB contamination. It is one of at least four major Anniston-related lawsuits against Monsanto and Solutia that have been filed by a total of 25,000 plaintiffs. Two of the cases have already been settled for a combined $80 million.

> In the first two weeks of testimony, the plaintiff's lawyers have established through Monsanto memorandums [sic] that the company was aware of the level of its discharges and that it at least partly understood the risks as early as the mid-1960s, if not earlier…A witness for the plaintiffs testified…that PCB levels in the blood of many plaintiffs was elevated. The 16 plaintiffs in

the first phase of the trial had average PCB levels of 46 parts per billion, 27 times the national norm, said Dr. Ian Nisbet, a Massachusetts toxicologist...

A 1966 letter by a Mississippi State University scientist who was hired by the company to test creek water disclosed that 25 fish, when submerged in Snow Creek, 'lost equilibrium and turned on their sides in 10 seconds and were dead in three and a half minutes.[13]

Unfortunately, this Monsanto example is only one in thousands of cases of known chemical dumping that has led to cancer, deaths, disease and other risks and problems in the United States and beyond. The destruction of our environment by chemicals is leading to our demise because as human organisms, we are tied to our environment and dependent on its bounty and its purity. The human body is not designed to cope with such chemicals, making disease probable and often fatal.

ARE WE LIVING NATURALLY OR ARTIFICIALLY?

It is often argued that people are living longer and healthier today than ever before in history. In response, we must ask the question: Who is telling us this? and Is it true? Perhaps drugs and modern medicine are keeping people alive for longer, but this is merely an artificial answer, not a natural, healthful approach. Just because people are surviving on drugs and cancer medications does not mean they are disease-free; nor does it mean that they are enjoying a rich quality of life. We must also credit increased sanitary conditions in our modern cities that have greatly improved the standard of living. Still, we cannot ignore that disease is still rampant in this modern era even among the affluent, if we stop to consider the ubiquitous chronic illness

---

13. Sack, Kevin, "PCB Pollution Suits Have Day in Court in Alabama," *The New York Times*, Sunday, Jan 27, 2002, page 18, National Report section

resultant from the modern, devitalized and chemicalized diet. We cannot ignore that the cancer rate continues to soar and that all of our cancer research has not even remotely begun to reverse or slow the tide of cancer.

If cancer is linked to chemical exposure and consumption, which has been proven in so many cases, then why does the cancer industry (associations, treatment centers, drug companies, etc.) continue to point to viruses and genetics as causative factors? Perhaps pointing the finger at the culprits—nuclear power plants, weapons manufacturers and chemical industries—is still taboo, as long as we live in a world wherein huge corporations continue to dictate how medical research is conducted as they dare not allow their own destructive activities to become public knowledge.

The lay person must keep in mind that scientific research is mostly funded by private corporations, not by our government, and not solely (if at all) for the benefit of our population. Rather, research is conducted to prove the value of drugs and modern medical treatment so that the chemicals, technologies and methodologies of modern medicine are well-accepted and selected as the preferred choice of treatment. Much research is, in fact, misguided, because certain research groups are in collusion with the cancer-causing chemical companies themselves. It has been reported that the American Cancer Society has a "three-decade track record of indifference and even hostility to cancer prevention. Examples include issuing a joint statement with the Chlorine Institute justifying the continued global use of persistent organochlorine pesticides, and also supporting the industry in trivializing dietary pesticide residues as avoidable risks of childhood cancer. ACS (American Cancer Society) policies are further exemplified by its allocation of less than 0.1 percent of its $700 million annual budget to environmental and occupational causes of cancer."[14] The American Cancer Society "has repeatedly refused to provide the scientific testimony congressional committees need to regulate occupational and environmental carcinogens [cancer-causing substances]."[15]

---

14. Phillips, Peter, *Censored 2001*, Seven Stories Press, New York, 2001, p. 145

15. ibid. p. 141

The American Cancer Society is just the tip of the iceberg, representing only one small part of the problem we face in the modern world with respect to understanding and acting upon those chemicals in our environment causing cancer, illness and death. Chemicals are not natural, and they wreak havoc on the human organism, creating a host of symptoms which modern medicine then treats with drugs and surgeries. This pattern cannot be broken until the general public wakes up to the problem of human-made chemicals in our environment and our food, then demands that irresponsible corporations cease their dangerous production and disposal.

What Can We Do?

We as consumers can refuse to buy products from companies that destroy our environment, give our children diseases and support destruction of natural resources to which we are akin and which we all need for sustenance and procreation. And, we can purchase and support products and companies that truly promote health for us and the earth. Although it is rare that we hear of such companies in the mainstream media, they exist in the thousands in the United States and can be found on the Internet. Further, letter-writing, email and lobbying efforts have an impact. Communities across American have successfully fought industry polluters and forced them to stop poisoning their water, air and food supplies. It takes work and commitment, but this is a fight for your life.

At the conclusion of his report on Kids & Chemicals, Bill Moyers advises, "…even when the science is sound and the laws are in place it's up to the community to get results."[16]

BACK TO THE NATURALIST PHILOSOPHY

Having taken a very brief look at three of the main causes of disease in this modern world, we can readily see that only one of these causes—tempera-

---

[16]. NOW with Bill Moyers, PBS transcript, May 10, 2002.

ture extremes—is really natural to human beings. The other two, which cause most of the illnesses in our world, are human-made and avoidable at the corporate level—corporations can refuse to produce and use dangerous and deadly chemicals and waste products—and the consumer level—we refuse to buy and use dangerous products.

You will note that listed among the few examples of man-made chemicals were vitamins. Although they cannot be compared to the horrific effects of toxic industrial chemicals, they are nevertheless chemicals capable of injuring the human body. If contained within their original foods, vitamins are supportive (helpful) substances; but once removed from their foods and/or created in a laboratory, vitamins have the potential of causing harm. Vitamins contained in foods are in balance; vitamins that are not contained in foods easily create imbalances.

Vitamins that are in pills and vitamin and multivitamin supplements **defy the naturalist philosophy.** Such substances never existed in primitive, ancient times, and they are not meant to be ingested any more than drugs are meant to be taken.

The only natural nutrients we can take are real, whole foods AND whole food concentrates, which be discussed in subsequent chapters. All other supplements are, by definition or design, NOT natural.

YOU ONLY HAVE TO REMEMBER THIS ONE POINT

All you have to do to stay on Nature's path is remember one single fact. Even if you do not read another page of this book, this one point will be enough to know in determining the goodness of vitamins and other supplements: **Nutrients are only natural if they are <u>still contained within</u> their original foods; human beings are meant <u>only</u> to ingest (eat) natural nutrients. Singular vitamins or minerals or amino acids (even if grouped together within the same supplement) do not qualify as natural; neither do human-made chemicals.**

SYNERGISM: THE SECRET TO STRENGTH & HEALING

It's right there in all of our notable clichés, but nobody pays attention: *There's strength in numbers...United we stand...Let's work together...A chain is as strong as its weakest link...Join hands...Two heads are better than one...The sum is only as good as its parts...*etc. These old adages are telling us that strength and success comes from combining the effort of each individual with that of other individuals; it's the undeniable power of teamwork and synergy. So how do we apply this concept to health and nutrition?

The power and healing virtues of foods lie not just in their nutrients, but rather in their innumerable parts working together as a team to feed, protect and enable our cells to carry on their functions. Food nutrients and other food substances **work together** for the greater cause! This is their secret to healing—the secret "ingredient" that continues to elude scientists. And this is why we cannot live on vitamin and mineral pills alone. The interwoven, interrelated and complementary functions of food particles represent some of Nature's most wonderful properties of **synergistic power and function.**

Synergism is defined as "the interaction of two or more agents or forces so that their combined effect is greater than the sum of their individual effects; working together."[17] Synergism explains how foods work to keep us healthy—promoting vibrance, healing, energy, creativity and even

---

17. American Heritage Dictionary, 4th Edition, p. 832

enjoyment of life. Synergism explains how calcium needs vitamin C and vitamin A and essential fatty acids to be effective; and synergism explains how bioflavonoids work together with vitamin C and proteins and minerals to strengthen the blood vessels. The synergistic nature of food cannot be recreated by scientists; it is too complex, and it contains the intangible, ever-present element we call "life energy."

What gives living beings, including plants, animals and humans, "life"? This is an eternal question that is more often addressed by religious leaders or philosophers than scientists, probably because, despite their eye-opening discoveries ABOUT life, they still do not have a clue as to the missing link that IS life. This is an eternal mystery, yet the modern medical industry continues to ignore the reality that Nature's whole foods are so powerful, precise and balanced in their healing and health-promoting properties because they, unlike drugs and vitamin pills, are LIVING and brimming with synergistic factors too numerous and too complex to duplicate in a laboratory.

We can survive on real foods, but we will surely suffer and die consuming too many, or the wrong kinds of, drugs and vitamin pills. Living things, such as the plants and animals we eat, contain interactive ingredients (nutrients) that work together like keys to unlock the doors to our cells. Other such ingredients deliver nutrients directly into our cells, while still other nutrients feed our cells the building blocks of health, energy, protection and activity. As living entities, we humans thrive in bodies that recognize Nature's foods as harmonious, helpful, complex, useful and beneficial substances. On the other hand, our bodies do not recognize drugs and vitamin pills—both known as "chemicals"—as "friendly" or complete. This is proven by the way our bodies respond to the introduction of chemicals. Doctors and researchers refer to the response as *side effects*.

Isolated chemicals, such as drugs and singular vitamins, are regarded by our bodies as foreign invaders. Therefore, when consumed, our bodies react by trying to oust the chemicals as quickly as possible, producing symptoms such as perspiration, rapid heartbeat, heavier breathing, fever, nausea, liver congestion, skin rashes, mucous build-up and more. If allowed to stay in our bodies, more serious side effects are caused, including digestive problems, serious skin conditions, headaches, fever, flu-like symptoms, degeneration of tissue, internal bleeding, damage to blood vessels and the heart, liver and kidney disease, chronic respiratory illness and much more. Side effects are Nature's way of telling us that certain substances do not belong in our bodies.

To be fair, we must also say that some natural substances can cause side effects and symptoms too; but in this context of health-promotion, we are talking about substances that we purposefully take to enhance, support and promote our health—which is supposed to be the point of taking vitamins and drugs. Allergies to foods is a whole other topic and frequently has much more to do with weakened immune systems and other such complications than the fault of a natural, unaltered food. In other words, if you eat a good, wholesome, nourishing food, then suffer from allergic reactions, the real problem may be more with your own body than with the food itself. Conversely, if you take drugs and vitamin pills then get sick, you can be assured that these are not natural substances and your body is not meant to tolerate them.

As we shall see, drugs and vitamin pills are merely chemicals and contain none of Nature's inherent synergists that make foods so special in the healing and prevention picture. It is the complexity of food substances—from nutrients to vitamins, and from carbohydrates to plant pigments—that makes food a natural healer. This complexity is based on a system of synergism that has no equal in our human-made medical arsenal. The concept of "getting back to nature," then, takes on a powerfully charged meaning as we look at foods for health and recovery. Each food nutrient and substance works together in infinite ways and combinations to harmonize with our own biochemistry and physiology, feeding billions of dynamic, busy cells so they can perform their life-promoting activities.

Health and vitality is a complex system, not a simplistic one. This explains why, when we use drugs or isolated vitamin substances, we easily create a biochemical imbalance by disturbing the natural synergism that directs and creates life, health and healing. By adding one drug to our system, we can create a chain reaction of adverse cellular functions, trading one health problem for another. By introducing one single mineral or a small number of minerals to our bodies, we can create a domino effect of internal events that endanger our health. In accord with the naturalist/wholistic philosophy, we should leave healing to the innate intelligence and synergy of Nature's foods.

WHAT IS A VITAMIN
WITHOUT OTHER NUTRIENTS?

Much has been written about what a vitamin IS, but not much has been said about vitamins that still exist within the context of the entire food wherein they are found. Therefore, people are more apt to speak about vitamins as isolated, independent, individual chemicals rather than (and more importantly) how vitamins interact and interrelate with other substances found alongside them within the whole food complex. By analogy, we can speak of a human heart and its function, but we must never forget that a heart is only as good as the rest of the body's organs, tissues and nerve impulses. A heart by itself is not a living entity—it must have the rest of the body to be meaningful, functional and valuable. By the same notion, as shall be repeated perhaps too often in this book, a vitamin never exists alone (in isolation) in a food, but rather alongside of, and interwoven with, other nutrients and substances that all work together to support our cells. Doctors and patients alike tend to ignore the fact that there are many, many other nutrients, substances and properties within foods that are just as important as vitamins, and that help vitamins work. Metaphorically speaking, a roof is very important for keeping out the rain and no other structure accomplishes this unique task, but we have to admit that the roof could not function without walls and a foundation. Without other food substances, then, vitamins are just chemicals, like drugs. And we cannot live on isolated vitamins without the other food properties our cells need to keep us in a state of health, balance and vitality.

The Vitamin Discovery

In 1912, a Polish chemist named Casimir Funk, proposed that disease may be caused by a missing ingredient that should be in the diet. He suggested that this ingredient was responsible for giving life (*vita*) and contained nitrogen (*amine*). Although not all vitamins contain nitrogen, the word "vitamin" has survived since its naming by Funk who set in motion the idea that many diseases may be cured by administering foods rich in certain vitamins.

Vitamin by Definition

A vitamin is defined as "a general term for a number of unrelated organic [containing carbon and come from living materials such as plants and animals; or that were once living] substances that occur in many foods in small amounts and that are necessary in trace amounts for the normal metabolic functioning of the body. They may be water-soluble or fat soluble."[18] That's the medical textbook definition. Now in plain English. A vitamin is a part of a food that never exists alone—by itself (in isolation)—but rather within a food, and in small amounts, to help the body's cells work in health and vitality. There is no such thing as a vitamin tree or a vitamin bush or a vitamin berry, because vitamins are not foods; they are only **parts** of foods and they, according to medical books, are not meant to be consumed in large quantities in the diet; they do not occur in "megadose" quantities within any of Nature's foods. Vitamins are "substances which, in small amounts, are necessary to sustain life. They must be obtained from food as they are either not made in the body at all, or are not made in sufficient quantities for growth, vitality and well-being. Lack of a particular vitamin or mineral can lead to incomplete metabolism, fatigue and other health problems; and in severe cases, to deficiency disease."[19]

---

18. *Dorland's Illustrated Medical Dictionary*, 26th Edition, W.B. Saunders Company, Philadelphia, 1985, p.1462

19. Reavley, Nicola, *The New Encyclopedia of Vitamins, Minerals, Supplements & Herbs*, M. Evans & Company, New York, 1998, p.3

Popularity of Vitamins

Maybe a hundred years ago very few people knew about vitamins, but today the word "vitamin" is a household word. The vitamin's popularity comes from the marketing success of chemical companies that have promoted the use of vitamins just as they have succeeded in promoting the use of drugs as wonder pills and cure-alls. But we now know better than to accept the cure-all philosophy. Or do we?

"Vitamin and mineral supplement sales are a $6.4 billion market; herbal supplements bring in at least $1.2 billion. The most dramatic increase in sales has occurred in the use of single vitamin supplements such as vitamin C, E, calcium and antioxidant tablets. The FDA reports that 53 percent of adults, or 101 million Americans, take nutritional supplements, with about 58 percent of women and 47 percent of men using vitamins or minerals. Typical users have some college education and fall in the middle to upper income range."[20]

LOOKING FOR SPECTACULAR RESULTS WITH VITAMIN PILLS

What do people expect to achieve by eating vitamin pills? Because most people are not very informed about how vitamins are made and what they are capable—and not capable—of doing, they rely on marketing claims. Like all marketing claims, some of what is said about vitamins is true and other statements are false; still other claims are misguided and misleading. It is true that vitamins are PARTS of foods, but they are NOT foods. It is true that **foods contain vitamins**, but it is not necessarily true that the vitamins you take are actually FROM foods (vitamins can also be made synthetically in a laboratory just as drugs are manufactured). And it is true that NO vitamin is really "natural" once it has been REMOVED from its original source—the food that once contained the vitamin.

---

20. Shayne, Ph.D., Vic, *Whole Food Nutrition: The Missing Link in Vitamin Therapy*, iuniverse, Lincoln, NE, 2001, p.12

WE NEED MUCH MORE THAN JUST VITAMINS FOR HEALTH & PREVENTION

Not long ago, when the vitamin craze hit America, the modern medical community made a very strong statement against the use of vitamins and other supplements. They told us that these supplements were dangerous, bad for us, unnecessary and part of an overall system of quackery. Critics of modern medicine claimed these harsh condemnations were expressions of fear. The medical establishment was afraid—and still is—that alternative, or natural, health care was infringing on the medical institution's money-making, monopolistic enterprise. The thought that people could take health care into their own hands was a horrifying one that threatened the medical community in the most sensitive area—the pocketbook. The only way to get people to stop buying vitamins, herbs, minerals and other supplements, and to prevent them from seeking out alternative therapies to drug and surgical approaches, was to launch an all-out defamation campaign, telling us through every major media that vitamins and herbs are dangerous and even deadly. In this wake, by the way, the medical establishment ignored the fact that modern medical procedures and drugs are far more dangerous and deadly, and there are statistics to prove this fact. The attack on the alternative health and supplement industries has changed course over the last ten years only because major drug companies are now producing many of the vitamin supplements on the market today. They couldn't beat 'em, so they joined 'em. Now the attack is focused mainly on natural health care modalities and practitioners—naturopaths, nutritionists, Chinese medical doctors, chiropractors, acupuncturists and others who offer a more natural approach to health care.

At one point, the modern medical community exclaimed that we did not need supplements because we could get "all of the vitamins and minerals we needed in our daily diet." We don't hear this claim very much any more, and maybe it's too bad because there is a hint of validity in this—at least theoretically. Yes, foods can provide important nutrients, and in a better form and balance than exists in vitamin pills. However, the fundamental problem with the aforementioned statement is that today's diets are fail to offer health, immunity, prevention and nutritional value. Today's diets are full of chemicals, preservatives, dead foods, altered fats and other foul nutrition. In addition, today's foods lack nutrients, including vitamins, minerals, enzymes, essential fatty acids and other properties that our bodies desperately need to function optimally. Theoretically, we should get our vitamins and minerals from our diets; and our diets should really contain natural, whole foods like alfalfa, wheat bran, carrots, broccoli, spinach, apples, oranges, good meats, nuts, seeds, berries and more— all uncooked and unprocessed. Vitamin, mineral and multivitamin supplements do not contain the nutrients that exist within such foods. You can, however, find them in a whole food concentrate supplement—a supplement comprised of whole, raw foods that have been concentrated into tablet, powder or capsule form. Yet, we must always keep in mind that even whole food concentrates are still supplements—not *replacements* for foods, but rather *additions* to a sound and healthful diet that is made up of a variety of natural foods.

Foods contain a plethora of nutrients and substances not found in vitamin pills, multivitamin supplements or mineral supplements. An apple, for instance, contains a skin that helps clean the intestinal (digestive) tract, a juicy meat full of many vitamins, minerals, enzymes and natural sugars, and an easy-to-digest juice that is chock full of nutrients. If you bite into a vitamin pill, I guarantee it is not as delicious as an apple. That's because a vitamin is not a food. An apple a day is said to keep the doctor away, but a vitamin pill cannot make the same claim. Why not? A vitamin pill is incomplete; it's missing the wonderful, mouthwatering, nutritious, fiber-filled and substantive traits of the apple.

Whole Food Concentrates

Whole food concentrates, which are actually real, whole foods (such as broccoli, spinach, liver, beets, etc.) that have been concentrated into tablet, powder or capsule form, are the best type of supplement available, as opposed to vitamin and multivitamin pills. Whole food concentrates contain a wide array of nutrients and other food constituents (parts) that are not to be found in other types of supplements—especially not vitamin or mineral or multivitamin pills (see illustration below). Vitamins, minerals, amino acids and enzymes are only **parts** of foods, they are not foods themselves; they are incomplete. By analogy, we can say that a steering wheel is a part of a car, but without the rest of the automobile, we cannot drive with only a steering wheel. Or, we can say that a hand is a natural part of the body, but we know that a hand without the rest of the body's parts, both large and small, can no longer function. To take this comparison one step further, you cannot remove a hand from a body then mix it in a box with other body parts and expect that it will still function, even though, chemically speaking, it may still have the same natural composition as any other hand. Similarly, then, even if you remove a vitamin from a food and call it "natural," you cannot simply mix it back in with other foods and expect it to still function as a real food. A vitamin that is not still contained within its original food is nothing more than just a CHEMICAL, no longer sharing its synergistic relationships.

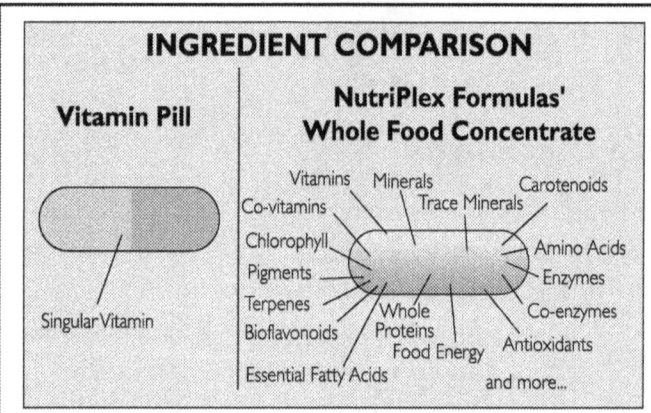

INGREDIENT COMPARISON

Vitamin Pill

**NutriPlex Formulas'
Whole Food Concentrate**

Singular Vitamin

Vitamins   Minerals   Carotenoids
Co-vitamins   Trace Minerals
Chlorophyll   Amino Acids
Pigments   Enzymes
Terpenes   Whole   Co-enzymes
Bioflavonoids   Proteins
                Food Energy   Antioxidants
Essential Fatty Acids   and more...

This simple chart shows the comparison between a vitamin pill
vs. a whole food concentrate supplement. The pill is an "isolate,"
meaning that it contains only a vitamin, such as vitamin A
Palmitate or vitamin C ascorbic acid. The food concentrate, on
the other hand, contains not only the vitamin, but also a host of
other nutrients indigenous to the food as found in nature. Thus,
foods are said to be "complex," meaning that they contain a
wide array of different, interactive, interwoven and dynamic
substances balanced in nature's foods. Human beings cannot
survive on vitamins alone.

Courtesy ©2002 NutriPlex Formulas, Inc.,
www.nutriplexformulas.com

Vitamins in Isolation are Just Chemicals

Vitamin supplements may contain one, two or many different vitamins, but these vitamins are not the same as vitamins that are **still contained** within their original foods. Beyond this concept, vitamins that are *synthetic* are created in a laboratory like drugs, and are not natural even in the most remote sense. A synthetic vitamin is like a silk plant. It may look like a real plant, take up the same amount of space, be pleasing to the eye, collect dust in the same way and serve some of the same aesthetic functions, but it is not natural, nor is it alive, nor was it ever alive.

Vitamin C ascorbic acid is a good example of a synthetic vitamin because it is manufactured not in nature, but in a laboratory, from corn sugar. If you buy vitamin C ascorbic acid pills, you should know that it does not come from oranges and lemons or any other fruit. Vitamin manufacturers like to show us images of oranges and lemons, but you can be certain that vitamin C ascorbic acid supplements are not foods and are not natural. They work as drugs in the body, not as complete, complex food nutrients even though they may look and act with some shared similarities.

THE CELLULAR LEVEL

There are trillions of cells inside and outside our bodies that carry on a seemingly infinite number of functions. Some cells comprise our nervous system, some make up our skin; some form our glands; and many others carry on very specific tasks. Cells are active—they reproduce, move around, exchange information with one another, protect us with immune functions; form protective barriers; knit damaged tissue back together; and perform other important tasks. Some cells are blood cells, others are liver cells and still others are brain cells. Cells perform as teams because they depend upon one another for success in promoting good health and healing. Every part of our bodies is made up of cells.

For our cells to work and do their jobs to their greatest ability and potential, they need nutrients. Nutrients come from the foods we eat, the air we breathe, the water we drink and even the energy surrounding us. Some experts would argue that we even get important nourishment from love, acts of kindness, laughter and happy thoughts. Traditional Chinese Medicine teaches us that we also derive nourishment from unseen, universal energy called *chi* ("chee"). This concept gave birth to an ancient system of exercises—known as *Qi Gong*, or *Chi Kung*—to move chi through the body in an effort to continually stimulate every part of the body with life force, or energy. Ancient India founded a similar system—yoga—designed to increase the flow of energy throughout the body. Thus, the idea of nourishing our health is more than just a matter of nutrition, as it also incorporates various means of circulating energy, reducing stress, and improving one's mental and emotional states. Life is energy. Real, whole food is a source of living, natural energy; but vitamins in pills are not.

Vitamins and minerals alone are not enough to keep us alive and healthy. This is a fact of life. Although television ads, books, mail promotions and seminar speakers may try to sell us their vitamins, no doctor worth his salt will tell you that your body can thrive in health by consuming vitamins and minerals alone. This is why we need to eat real, whole foods. And when our diets are not complete enough, we may need to take whole food concentrates as well.

VITAMINS, MINERALS & AMINO ACIDS: IMPORTANT PARTS OF FOODS

A vitamin pill contains one or more vitamins. On the other hand, a real, whole, natural food (as well as a good quality whole food concentrate supplement) contains a host of wondrous, nutritious, life-supporting substances and qualities. Many of these are referred to as "phytonutrients" or "phytochemicals," which are biochemical substances that provide functions and contain properties that go far beyond the reach of vitamins and minerals. Phytochemicals, including known and unknown constituents of plants, feature flavonoids (of which there are thousands of types), phytoesterols, carotenoids, indoles, coumarins, organosulfur compounds, terpenes, saponins, lignans and isothiocyanates, to name but a few. Again, these substances are NEVER found in vitamin, multivitamin or mineral pills, but are contained in the natural complex of Nature's foods.

Here are some food substances—found in both whole food supplements, as well as whole, natural foods—and their roles:

Vitamins

Whole foods contain not just one, but several vitamins that interrelate and work together. For instance, in spinach you will find not just vitamin C, but also carotenes and folic acid. In real, whole foods, vitamins interact, often protecting one another from destruction. Vitamin C actually protects vitamin A within foods. And vitamin E keeps other vitamins from destruction due to exposure to oxygen. Vitamins also are found connected to *sub-vitamins*. For instance, most people have heard of vitamin A, but in Nature's whole foods, vitamin A is divided into several subgroups, such as vitamin A1 and vitamin A2, as well as retinols, retinoids and retinoic acid and essential fatty acids. Vitamins also works alongside minerals within foods. For example, in wheat germ, vitamin E works hand-in-hand with the mineral selenium; in liver, vitamin A carries on a relationship with zinc.

Minerals

Taber's Cyclopedic Medical Dictionary defines a mineral as "An inorganic element or compound occurring in nature, especially one that is solid. Minerals serve the following functions:

a. They are essential constituents of all cells

b. They form the greater portion of the hard parts of the body (bone, teeth, nails)

c. They are essential components of respiratory pigments, enzymes and enzyme systems

d. They regulate the permeability of cell membranes and capillaries

e. They regulate the excitability of muscular and nervous tissue

f. They are essential for regulation of osmotic pressure equilibria

g. They are necessary for maintenance of proper acid-base balance

h. They are essential constituents of secretions of glands

i. They play an important role in water metabolism and regulation of blood volume."[21]

---

21. *Taber's Cyclopedic Medical Dictionary 9th Ed.*, F.A. Davis Co. Philadelphia 1963, p. M41–M42

Minerals within foods are balanced by Nature, existing within a complex of other nutrients (including vitamins, as per previous examples) and other minerals. A single mineral, taken in a supplement by itself, has the potential to cause harm in our bodies because it may attract or carry away other minerals. For instance, too much magnesium or manganese interferes with the presence of calcium; too much iron will interfere with calcium levels; too much zinc upsets copper balance; too much phosphorus may unbalance calcium, etc. Foods do not contain only one mineral, but rather several within the complex. For instance, in parsley, you would find not only potassium, but also calcium, iron, selenium, phosphorus, magnesium, zinc and other minerals. Spinach, known as an iron food, also contains calcium, magnesium, phosphorus, selenium, copper, potassium, zinc and more, all in the same plant vegetable. Minerals that are not still contained within their original foods have a greater capacity for unbalancing vitamins as well. For instance, biochemists have found that too much copper will upset vitamin C levels in the body. The way minerals and vitamins are balanced is extremely complex and easy to unbalance through supplementation. Nature balances minerals in whole, natural foods.

Amino Acids

Proteins are made up of amino acids, which is why amino acids are called the "building blocks" of proteins. Amino acids and proteins are found in many types of plant and animal foods, including meats, glands, organs, seeds, cheese, milk, eggs, butter and beans. Nine of the 22 amino acids we need must be ingested in the foods we eat. These eleven are essential to receive through our diet; our bodies cannot manufacture them. Further, amino acids are not present in vitamin pills.

Without proteins we would literally fall apart and life would come to an immediate halt. The number of functions we owe to proteins would make your head spin, especially if you didn't have enough protein. Proteins carry on such tasks as keeping our skin together, digesting foods, creating hair and nails, regulating our hormonal system, building and rebuilding muscle, allowing chemical reactions to take place in our cells, etc.

There are many protein-builder and amino acid supplements on the shelves of health food stores these days; and such products are very much en vogue with athletes who believe they need amino acid "power shakes" to help build muscles and endurance. Both amateur and professional participants take isolated (and mixtures of isolated) amino acid supplements in an attempt to build and repair muscle that is damaged in the catabolism (breakdown) that takes place with exertion, injury, vigorous exercise and strenuous activity. In fact, athletes looking for the ultimate competitive edge share the common belief that they need huge amounts of protein in their diets to compensate for the stress created through their physical activity. Researchers, however, argue that excess protein, even in the face of heavy exertion, is unnecessary and potentially dangerous. Nutrition researchers at Tufts University conclude:

> To make their muscles bigger, bodybuilders often consume large quantities of protein, packing away huge amounts of meat and eggs and consuming protein drinks. But eating large amounts of protein does not build muscle; exercise, not diet, achieves that. As laboratory tests have shown, even animals on restricted diets will build muscles if they exercise.
>
> In the month before competition, many bodybuilders subsist on diets that consist almost entirely of protein. According to sports nutrition expert William Evans, this is a dangerous and ultimately self-defeating practice. Carbohydrate is needed to provide energy for the grueling daily regimen of exercise bodybuilders put themselves through. If muscle carbohydrate stores become depleted, which will occur on a low-carbohydrate diet, body builders will experience chronic fatigue.

Because eating disorders have lethal consequences, it is important that athletes and their trainers recognize the dangers of pushing the goal of achieving leanness beyond the point where it will ultimately harm performance.[22]

We should be aware that in nature's foods amino acids exist within a balanced environment and in small amounts. On the other hand, if you are taking amino acid supplements, there is a very great possibility of causing health problems.

Amino acid researchers Eric Braverman, M.D. and Carl Pfeiffer, M.D. caution: "Because many of the amino acids are absorbed and metabolized in a similar fashion, there is a great deal of competition between molecules. **Sometimes, one amino acid can cancel the effect of others.** This adds to the overall complexity of prescribing amino acids to treat disease. For example, amino acids compete for absorption with others in the same group, e.g., the aromatic amino acid group (tryptophan, tyrosine and phenylalanine) and can inhibit one another's passage into the brain."[23] To study the complex world of amino acids and their interactions, relationships and synergists, the reader is invited to study Dr. Braverman's, *The Healing Nutrients Within: Facts, Findings and New Research on Amino Acids* (Keats Publishing, 1987).

Another popular notion is that because protein is needed for the development of muscle, a high-protein diet will make a person muscular. These ideas are unproven, or at least gross oversimplifications that can lead to trouble when people take them literally. As eagerly as we might seek "magical" effects from food, the simple

---

[22.] Gershoff, Ph.D., Stanley, *The Tufts University Guide to Total Nutrition*, Harper Perennial, NY 1996, page 315.

[23.] Braverman, M.D., Eric R. and Carl C. Pfeiffer, M.D., Ph.D., *The Healing Nutrients Within, Facts, Findings and New Research on Amino Acids,* Keats Publishing, New Canaan, Connecticut, 1987, pages 14–15.

fact remains that only by eating a balanced variety of foods can we get all the nutrients we need in the amounts we need them.

In fact, consuming an overabundance of protein can be expensive and inefficient. Our bodies are not able to store the amino acids they can't use, so the excess is used either for energy or converted to fat. Consider, too, that the waste products from excess protein metabolism are lost in the urine. Overconsumption can place a strain on the kidneys. Furthermore, the fat and cholesterol content of many high-protein foods can place you at risk for heart disease if you eat too much of them.

The amount of protein most people need is approximately 8 or 9 percent of their total calories, with needs being highest during periods of growth, such as childhood. For women who are pregnant or lactating, they are even higher. Americans consume an average of 12 to 14 percent of their calories in protein, yet we could eat even more—say 20 percent—and still be healthy.[24]

Protein, like carbohydrates and fats, should exist in balance within the diet. High protein (especially cooked protein) diets may lead to health complications such as kidney stones, acidity (leading to gout, arthritis, accumulation of uric acid and purines in the tissues, heart disease, etc.) The meat and potatoes diet, involving the consumption of large amounts of cooked meats at almost every meal, is said by many nutritionists to be the demise of modern man's health. Similarly, high protein diets to promote weight loss have come under fire by critics who warn that the dieter may be trading a slimmer body for kidney complications.

Although most of us think of meats, beans and legumes as the best sources of proteins, as we shall see throughout this study, the concept of "quantity" is often far less significant than "quality." This is illustrated in a

---

[24.] Gershoff, pages 7–10

recent finding reported by Eli Greenbaum of the Department of Energy's Oak Ridge National Laboratory in collaboration with researchers at the University of Southern California who have discovered a unique protein in spinach. Known as Photosystem One, this protein may be able to restore vision to people with macular degeneration and retina pigmentosis—two eye diseases that destroy photoreceptor activity in the eye. "Photosystem One generates electrical energy, which scientists hope can be used to trigger the function of light-receiving cells in the eye, restoring the retina's ability to perceive images."[25]

[25.] *Acres, USA*, "Health & Healing News," February 2002, page 35

WHAT DO VITAMINS DO?

Now that we have outlined the differences between isolated vitamins NOT contained within foods versus vitamins that exist as A PART OF whole foods, we can look at the individual roles of specific vitamins in foods. Always remember that we are engaging in this discussion to show how vitamins work WITHIN foods, not as chemical isolates. Just because we take a close look at individual vitamins, we cannot make the mistake of believing they work best as individual chemicals, because to do so would be to take vitamins out of their natural context. By analogy, just because we understand how a heart works does not suggest that the heart will work the same way once removed from the living organism. Certainly it will still be a heart, still look and feel like a heart and still maintain the same cellular and biochemical make-up, but we know without a doubt that it can no longer function naturally once removed from the complex that we call the whole human organism.

There are many excellent books that extoll the benefits and functions of vitamins, minerals and other food substances, so we will not go into great detail here. Rather, we offer a brief glance at the role of some of these substances so you can understand *their value and interrelationships within the natural foods* wherein they are found.

VITAMIN A

Most vitamin A in capsule form, sold to the public as "vitamin A," is in the form of the synthetic vitamin A palmitate. In the whole food form, however, vitamin A is an extremely complex substance. Those who take vitamin A (or even beta carotene) as a synthetic or isolated vitamin supplement are failing to ingest the rest of the entire complex needed to perform a continuous array of biochemical tasks needed for health, vitality and healing. Vitamin A, in its complete form, is found in animal foods and is especially high in liver.

"For thousands of years, liver has been used as a cure for night blindness but it was only in the early part of the 20th century that researchers discovered that it is a rich source of vitamin A, which is essential for healthy eyes. The first vitamin to be discovered, vitamin A was identified in 1913 when two American scientists showed that butter and egg yolk contained a substance which was necessary for healthy growth in rats. They called this substance 'fat soluble A.' (As with so many other food nutrients, despite the fact that vitamin A was the first vitamin to be discovered, its actions in the cells of our bodies are not well understood at a chemical level. However misunderstood how vitamins work at a biochemical level, it is the deficiency in specific vitamin-containing foods which makes their necessity and importance apparent.) By 1930 the structure of vitamin A was determined, and five years later it was found to be necessary for normal vision."[26]

Life on earth depends on vitamin A through its influence on shaping and creating specific cells as well as developing embryos; vitamin A is the nutrient that enables substances that eventually form into organs and limbs. In addition, parts of vitamin A, known as retinol and retinoic acid, are considered hormones of the steroid/thyroid hormone superfamily of proteins. (Vitamin D also acts in a similar capacity.) Hormones play a wide variety of roles in the development of living creatures, from defining sexual characteristics to providing energy, and more.[27]

Further, vitamin A functions in the synthesis (formation) of certain sugars and proteins necessary for mucous production and normal growth regulation.

[26.] American Society of Nutritional Science: Britton, G. (1995) *Structure and properties of carotenoids in relation to function.* FASEB J. 9: 1551–1558 ; and Krinsky, N.I. (1993) *Actions of carotenoids in biological systems.* Ann. Rev. Nutr. 13: 561–587.

[27.] ibid.

Vitamin A is necessary for the growth and repair of many body cells including those of bones, teeth, collagen and cartilage. It is also essential for *cell differentiation*, a "process whereby cells change to take on different structures and functions; for instance, when one cell becomes a liver cell, whereas another becomes a red blood cell. Vitamin A's role in cell differentiation is probably related to its ability to interact with a cell's DNA to turn on and off various cellular functions. The role of vitamin A in cell differentiation is important in the maintenance of epithelial tissue (the covering of internal and external surfaces of the body, including the lining of vessels and other small cavities), reproduction and immunity."[28]

Thus, vitamin A plays a central role in tissue development and maintenance. Deficiency of vitamin A may cause tissues of the membranes in the eyes, digestive tract, respiratory tract and genitourinary tract (esp. tissues of ovaries and testes) to harden and shrink. This hardening, known as *keratinization*, has been attributed to many types of diseases, including colds, pneumonia and so-called respiratory infections—all related to the drying out of membranes. Keratinization leads to scaliness of the skin, failure of growth in young animals, failure of reproduction and corneal opacity. Keratinization may cause eye dryness, with malfunction of tear ducts. Medical findings attribute *xerophthalmia* to vitamin A deficiency, a condition in which the cornea of the eye becomes cloudy and fails to allow light to pass through.

Vitamin A foods maintain differentiation of epithelial cells such as skin, lung, and intestinal tissue, but this form of vitamin A cannot be used in vision.[29]

---

28. Smolin, page 259.

29. Olson, J.A. (1994) *Vitamin A, retinoids, and carotenoids. In: Modern Nutrition in Health and Disease* (Shils, M.E., Olson, J.A. & Shike, M., eds), 8th ed., pp. 287–307, Lea & Febiger, Philadelphia, PA

Sporn, M.B., Roberts, A.B. & Goodman, D.S. (eds.) (1994) *The Retinoids*, 2nd ed. Raven Press, New York, NY.

Night blindness is an early symptom of vitamin A deficiency. The cause is said to be due to a lack of visual purple (rhodopsin) in the retina which depends on vitamin A for regeneration. Vitamin A is used by the eyes to convert the light-sensitive pigments of the retina used for vision.[30]

"It has been estimated that 0.5 million children in the world become blind each year; 70 percent of these are due to vitamin A deficiency. Over half of these blind children die from malnutrition and associated illnesses."[31]

Scientists claim that vitamin A is 'the anti-infective vitamin,' enabling body surfaces to act as barriers to invading micro-organisms and toxins. Biochemically, vitamin A stimulates and enhances many immune functions including antibody response and the activity of various white blood cells such as T helper cells and phagocytes (cells that get rid of dead and toxic cells). This immune-enhancing function is said to promote healing of infected tissues and increasing resistance to infection.

Vitamin A has antioxidant activity and plays a role in protecting against free radical damage (destruction of important oxygen-containing molecules in our bodies by toxic substances, pollution, etc.) contributing to many common diseases. Additionally, vitamin A is involved in how iron is used and stored within our bodies .

Because vitamin A is stored in the liver and is fat soluble, the presence of fat and bile in the intestines is necessary for vitamin A absorption. Vitamin A is joined to fatty acids in the intestinal lining, combined with other substances, and transported to the liver, where 90 percent of the body's vitamin A is stored. Ideally, around 80 to 90 percent of vitamin A in the diet is absorbed, although this is reduced in older people and those who have trouble absorbing fat, such as in pancreatitis, celiac disease and cystic fibrosis sufferers, who may run the risk of vitamin A deficiency.[32]

---

30. Guyton, M.D., Arthur C., *Function of the Human Body*, W. B. Saunders Company, Philadelphia, 1974

31. Olson.

32. ibid

Therefore, bile deficiency, often associated with liver and gall bladder problems, may lead to vitamin A deficiency. In this regard, isolated vitamin supplementation with fractionated or synthetic forms of vitamin A, without sufficient bile activity, may contribute to toxicity.

Vitamin A has long been a subject of study in regard to cancer treatment and prevention, especially in lung cancer, where the vitality of the cells lining the respiratory system is integral to health, immunity and function. In one five-year study culminating in 1981, reported by The National Academy of Sciences and involving 8,278 Norwegian men, intake of **foods with vitamin A activity** was associated with lower incidence of lung cancer independent of cigarette smoking. The same success was shared by a population of women in the 11-year follow up study and in hospital-based case-comparison studies in the United States and in England. Researchers in 1981 hypothesized that the relevant dietary exposure was with beta-carotene rather than retinol. This was subsequently supported by a 19-year prospective study of 1,954 middle-aged men in Chicago and population-based case-comparison studies in New Jersey, Hawaii and New Mexico. Two other studies—a 10-year prospective study of 265,118 adults in Japan and a hospital-based case-comparison study of Chinese subjects in Singapore—indicated that lung cancer risk was inversely associated with the frequency of eating green and yellow **vegetables.**[33]

Toxicity & Dangers of Vitamin A Supplements

Too much vitamin A can lead to liver disease as well as other problems. For a more complete study of the dangers of taking vitamin A supplements, please consult the author's book, *Whole Nutrition: The Missing Link in Vitamin Therapy* (2001), which cites a number of relevant scientific studies.

[33.] *Diet & Health, Implications for Reducing Chronic Disease Risk,* National Research Council, National Academy of Sciences, 1989, page 313.

Food Sources of Vitamin A

"While the vitamin A we obtain from food comes in many different forms, these can be divided into two main types—pre-formed vitamin A and provitamin A. Pre-formed vitamin A, which is often in the form of retinol or retinal, is found in foods of animal origin, such as liver and butter. Provitamin A is the name given to around 50 compounds in a group of plant pigments known as carotenes (or carotenoids), with beta carotene being the best known of these. This is because these compounds can be turned into vitamin A in the body. Both pre-formed vitamin A and provitamin A are fat soluble."[34]

Although beta carotene has been made very popular as a supplement, the fact is that there are more than 500 carotenoids in nature (some sources state there are more than 600 carotenoids). Carotenoids are efficient at absorbing light used for energy within plants and animals. They are also the major yellow and red pigments in many fruits and vegetables. Beta-carotene…and alpha-carotene are responsible for the orange color of carrots, and astaxanthin imparts a red or pink color to lobsters and salmon. Lycopene is responsible for the red color of tomatoes. Recent studies have shown that lycopene-rich foods fight cancer and protect immune cells:

> Lycopene found in tomatoes helps to protect against prostate cancer by shrinking tumors and slowing their spread, according to research presented at a meeting of the American Association for Cancer Research. Researchers from the Karmanos Cancer Institute in Detroit studied 33 men about to have surgery to remove cancerous prostate glands. For 30 days, they gave

---

34. American Society for Nutritional Sciences: Britton, G. (1995) *Structure and properties of carotenoids in relation to function. FASEB J.* 9: 1551–1558 ; and Krinsky, N.I. (1993) *Actions of carotenoids in biological systems. Ann. Rev. Nutr.* 13: 561–587.

lycopene capsules to half of the men and placebo to the others. The results showed that cancer tissue was less likely to extend clear to the edges of the prostate glands of those who had used lycopene. The pre-cancerous cells in their prostates were less abnormal looking. The amount of lycopene taken was similar to the amount found in about a pound of tomatoes. However, since lycopene is not easily absorbed from raw tomatoes, a person may need to eat two to three pounds to raise blood levels as high as that seen in the study.

In another study, published in the *American Journal of Clinical Nutrition,* researchers found that women who ate a diet containing tomatoes had less free radical damage to the white blood cells of their immune systems than those who ate a tomato-free diet.[35]

Biochemically speaking, the term "carotene" refers to carotenoids which contain only carbon and hydrogen (e.g. beta-carotene, alpha-carotene, lycopene), while the term "xanthophylls" refers to compounds which contain hydroxyl groups (lutein, zeaxanthin, beta-cryptoxanthin) or keto groups (canthaxanthin) or both (astaxanthin).

Vitamin A is found in liver, fish liver oils, butter, milk and (to a lesser extent) in kidneys, fat and muscle meats. Vitamin A occurs naturally only in foods of animal origin, but the body converts certain carotenoids, especially beta carotene, to vitamin A. Only 50 of the more than 500 naturally occurring carotenoids have provitamin A activity. Provitamin A is a precursor (building block) of vitamin A and is found in yellow fruits and vegetables including peaches, carrots, apricots, squash, and sweet potatoes. Provitamin A can be converted into vitamin A within the body. As with any vitamin found in its original food complex, vitamin A is made up of

---

35. American Journal of Clinical Nutrition 1999:69:712–718

several different components and is made to work as a nutrient not only by being intact with its other components, but also as it exists alongside other nutrients (minerals such as zinc and iron, trace mineral activators, enzymes, etc.). Vitamin A is a family of compounds that includes retinol, retinal and the carotenoids. Therefore, it is important to consider that vitamin A is not an isolated substance, but rather "the name given to **a group of compounds** which have certain actions in the body."[36]

VITAMIN B COMPLEX

The vitamin B complex is perhaps one of the most overlooked nutrient groups which, when lacking in the diet, leads to deficiencies that cause a great number of so-called diseases and "vague" symptoms. The first of the vitamin B complex to be discovered was vitamin B1 (thiamine) in 1926. However, vitamin B1's notoriety grew worldwide when it was found, as an ingredient in brown rice, to be effective in treating the disease called *beriberi*, rampant amongst American prisoners of war in both World War II and in the Korean War. Characterized by extreme fatigue and mental distress, beriberi was once thought to be caused by germs until it was discovered that prisoners of war were being fed polished rice that had been stripped of its vitamin B value.

In the case of vitamin B deficiency, nearly every cell in the body is affected. B vitamins are needed for the production and release of energy in every cell, and no cell can do its work without energy. Symptoms of B vitamin deficiencies include nausea, severe exhaustion, irritability, depression, forgetfulness, loss of appetite and weight, pain in muscles, impairment of the immune response, loss of control of the limbs, abnormal heart action, severe skin problems, teary or bloodshot eyes, and many more (irregular heartbeat, anemia, enlarged heart, blood cell damage, cracks in the sides of the mouth, digestive disturbances, swollen tongue, brain damage, chronic fatigue, paranoia, attention deficit).

---

36. ibid.

"Because cell renewal depends on energy, protein and DNA/RNA availability, and because all of these depend on the B vitamins, tissues in which the cells' life spans are shortest are most readily damaged by B vitamin deficiency."[37]

Jack Cooperman, Ph.D., director of nutrition at New York Medical College states, "It takes only a few weeks for the [vitamin] B levels in your blood to drop. This increases the risk of a subclinical deficiency, which can occur after active forms of the B vitamins in the cells decrease."[38]

Despite the subclinical (not yet detectable by scientific tests or doctor examination), symptomatic evidence of vitamin B deficiency, as of this writing, the standard consensus amongst the scientific community is that vitamin B deficiency is rare in this day and age of mass enrichment and fortification of foods. However, because enrichment is performed with synthetic (isolated) vitamins, it appears that such synthetic use of vitamin B fails to provide the body with what it needs to achieve optimal health. Food-based vitamin B (natural foods that contain B vitamins, such as yeast, wheat germ, whole rice, etc.), on the other hand, is found along with important cofactors (helper nutrients) within the same whole foods that enable B vitamins to be used by our bodies as nutrients for a great number of functions.

The B vitamins are often found together in food and were first thought as a single substance needed to produce energy from food. They are now described to be eight individual nutrients with separate functions required for various steps in the use of carbohydrates, proteins and fats. "The B vitamins also interact; some are needed to convert others into their active...forms, and a deficiency of any one can interfere with energy metabolism and cause some common deficiency symptoms. For example, depression and weakness may result from a deficiency of one or more of the B vitamins."[39]

[37.] Hamilton, page 206.

[38.] Faelten, Sharon, Ed., *The Complete Book of Vitamins and Minerals*, Rodale Press, Inc., New Jersey, 1988, page 92.

[39.] Smolin, page 280.

Nutrition researcher Joan Priestly, M.D. and health editor Carolyn Reuben agree: "if you take a disproportionately large dose of one B vitamin, after a few weeks the body will begin to complain with myriad distress symptoms. It needs the other Bs to use any one of them effectively."[40]

"In academic discussions of the vitamins, clearly different deficiency symptoms are given for each one. Actually such clear-cut symptoms are found only in laboratory animals that have been fed contrived diets that lack just one ingredient. In real life, a deficiency of any one B vitamin seldom shows up by mixtures of nutrients. Still the deficiency of one B vitamin may appear predominant in a cluster of deficiencies, and often, if it is corrected by giving **wholesome food rather than single supplements**, the subtler deficiencies will be corrected along with it."[41]

As each vitamin B was discovered, it was given a number to distinguish it from the other B vitamins in the family. Some substances that were once thought to be B vitamins also were entitled with a special number, then later, after research revealed that the substance was not really a vitamin, the number was dropped from the series. This is why, for instance, there is no vitamin B4 or B7-11. Vitamin B complex contains these individual B vitamins that act together as co-workers: thiamine (B1), riboflavin (B2), niacin (B3), pantothenic acid (B5), pyridoxine (B6), cobalamin (B12).

B vitamins are found in a number of natural foods, but have been mostly stripped away from the most common foods that are part of today's modern diet. For instance, in food processing, vitamin B is destroyed by heat and milling. One of the richest sources of some of the B vitamins is in the germ of wheat, within the oily portions of the plant. However, food processors remove the germ of the plant, and the oils, because these portions of the plant are apt to have a very short shelf life before they begin to spoil. By removing the vitamin B from the plant, processed foods last

---

40. Reuben, page 135.

41. Hamilton, page 208.

longer, making profits higher. It is therefore a consideration of business, not nutrition, that vitamin B is stripped from most foods. Manufacturers of processed, refined food products have subsequently tried to make up for the loss in vitamin B by "enriching" their foods, including bread and flour products. However, enrichment involves the use of synthetic, isolated vitamin B, not the original complex food version of the entire vitamin B complex. This is why many researchers feel that a vitamin B deficiency is not only likely, but *probable*, in our modern world even though government, medical and corporate officials claim that vitamin B is present in foods (through artificial enrichment) and that deficiencies are rare.

One of the greatest symptoms of vitamin B deficiency is now labeled chronic fatigue syndrome, a condition wherein people feel tired, depressed, without motivation and generally run down. Since vitamin B is responsible for producing energy in the body's cells (among thousands of other roles), chronic fatigue (and many other associated symptoms) is not surprising in this age of processed, dead food diets.

Other B Vitamin Deficiency Problems

Recent research (as of 1999) shows that vitamin B_{12} deficiency "may increase the risk of neural tube defects in pregnant women with a high risk of this condition. Vitamin B_{12} deficiency may be common in AIDS and also in developing countries, probably due to malabsorption combined with low intakes."[42]

In addition, according to one study at the University of Georgia (1999), low levels of B vitamins were found to cause hearing impairment. More specifically, in a small study of 55 healthy women ages 60 to 71, vitamin B_{12} and folate were linked to hearing loss. In this group, women with damaged hearing had 38 percent lower vitamin B_{12} and 31 percent lower red cell folate than women with normal hearing.[43]

---

42. ibid.

43. *American Journal of Clinical Nutrition*, 1999; 69; 564–571.

Foods Containing B Vitamins

Vitamin B is available from the diet through a variety of whole foods. Among these are wheat germ, rice, yeast, grains and seeds, organ meats (liver and kidney), bivalve mollusks (clams and oysters), poultry, egg yolks, fermented cheeses and dry milk. Algae such as nori and spirulina contain vitamin B_{12} analogs that are argued to be biologically inactive in humans. Animal and fish muscle contain very small amounts of vitamin B_{12}.

VITAMIN C

Some natural health care doctors insist food sources of vitamin C achieve NUTRITIVE results, whereas synthetic isolated ascorbic acid vitamin C (the kind sold as vitamin C supplements, made from corn sugar) contributes only to a pharmacological (drug-like) effect.

Yet, natural health care doctor or not, all experts agree that **any vitamin in an isolated form requires at least the presence of certain cofactors (helper nutrients) for it to work.** When you consume an isolated vitamin, the body must provide the cofactors for that vitamin to work. When you consume a food containing vitamins and other nutrients, the same food also provides necessary cofactors so your body is not forced to compensate for the burden. Over time, taking isolated vitamins may very possibly lead to any one of a number of deficiencies as the body must continually surrender its stores of cofactors (including certain enzymes, proteins, minerals, essential fats, helper vitamins, etc.) in order to make the *isolated* vitamins (such as vitamin C ascorbic acid supplements) work.

Much of the publicity about the benefits and effects of vitamin C come from the work of Dr. Linus Pauling. Pauling became adamant in his claims that vitamin C is perhaps the most important nutrient needed in the diet and he advocated taking megadoses, ranging from one to 10 grams (10,000 milligrams) per day and up. Compare this amount to the recommended daily dietary dosage of between 60mg to 200mg. Such high dosages of vitamin C recommended by Pauling, of course, does not equate

to nutrition, but rather to chemical use—pharmacology. Pauling did wonders for the vitamin industry's sales, but what is the health effect on consumers? We'll probably never know, especially since the effects of high
dosage vitamins in many cases are not immediately noticed. They may
affect the consumer by creating a series of biochemical chain reactions
producing any one of myriad deficiencies and symptoms that would be
difficult to trace directly back to the effects of megadosing. Because the
human biochemistry is a delicate system that depends on balance in a
dynamic (ever-changing) environment, it is folly to believe that high
dosages of ANY substance will not eventually cause a health problem, no
matter how safe any scientist or company claims their product is.

Author Elson M. Haas, M.D. writes, "Overall, it is probably best to
take vitamin C as it is found in nature, along with the vitamin P constituents—the bioflavonoids, rutin, and hesperidin. These may have a
synergistic influence on the functions of vitamin C…"

Haas continues:

> In recent years, the _C_ of this much-publicized vitamin has…stood
> for _C_ontroversy. With Linus Pauling and others claiming that vita-
> min C has the potential to prevent and treat the common cold,
> flu, and cancer, all of which plague our society, concern has arisen
> in the medical establishment about these claims and the megadose
> requirements needed to achieve the hoped-for results. Some stud-
> ies suggest that these claims have some validity; however, there is
> more personal testimony from avid users of ascorbic acid than
> there is irrefutable evidence. '_C_' also stands for citrus, where this
> vitamin is found [although vitamin C supplements are not made
> from citrus, but rather from corn sugar]. It could also stand for
> collagen, the protein 'cement' that is formed with ascorbic acid as
> a required cofactor. Many foods contain vitamin C, and many
> important functions are mediated by it as well.[44]

---

44. Haas

Vitamin C Deficiency

Like any other vitamin provided by nature, vitamin C is very important to life and health. Vitamin C deficiency, the symptoms of which were once considered the result of a contagious disease, has been the archenemy of armies, navies and explorers throughout history. A vitamin C deficiency could wipe out a ship of sailors more effectively and tragically than a war at sea.

Known as *scurvy*, vitamin C deficiency was described by ancient peoples, most notably those who spent considerable time at sea and away from fresh, vitamin-C bearing foods. Greeks, Egyptians and Romans made note of the ravages of this seemingly uncontrollable disease from as early as 1500 B.C. Aristotle describes the illness in 450 B.C. "as a syndrome characterized by lack of energy, gum inflammation, tooth decay, and bleeding problems. "[45] We now know this disease as *scurvy*.

Unenlightened medical pundits at the time blamed vitamin C deficiency disease on all sorts of off-base causations, ranging from demonic possession to heresy, and from bad blood to a contagion demanding quarantine. However, astute observers of the day began to note a relation between scurvy and a lack of certain foods, which later scientists identified as vitamin C-bearing foods. But new, life-enhancing ideas were slow to be to accepted by conservative purveyors of "modern" medicine...

> In the mid-1500s the Indians of eastern Canada knew that an extract from white cedar needles would cure the disease (scurvy). An association between citrus fruit and scurvy was first noted in the 16th century when Sir Richard Hawkins observed on his voyage to the South Seas that the sickness could be cured by oranges and lemons. Despite his observation, 10,000 British soldiers died of scurvy that same year. [It was difficult at that time, as it remains, to convince the established medical system to change their way of thinking to accept nutritional explanations for diseases and symptoms]. Over 100 years later, James Lind, a

---

[45.] ibid.

Scottish physician serving the British navy, tested various agents for their effectiveness at curing scurvy and reported that two patients given citrus fruits recovered within six days. Despite his study, it was another 48 years before the passage of the Merchant Seaman's Act of 1835 which required that lime or lemon juice be included in the rations of the mercantile service and earned British sailors the name *limeys*."[46]

Without vitamin C foods, the tissues of the body become "unglued," so to speak. This is the trademark of scurvy—the undoing of tissues that leads to bleeding and eventually death. Scurvy is characterized by easily bruised skin, muscle fatigue, soft swollen gums, decreased wound healing and hemorrhaging, osteoporosis and anemia. These symptoms exist today even among modern peoples, especially those whose diets are largely based on cooked, processed and denatured foods.

Essential to collagen (cells that hold other cells together) formation, vitamin C helps maintain the integrity of connective tissue as well as the blood and lymphatic vessels. This includes skin tissue, osteoid tissue of bone and dentin of teeth. Vitamin C also participates in the creation of folic acid, absorption of iron and metabolism of amino acids such as *phenylalanine* (essential for optimal growth in infants and for nitrogen equilibrium in human adults) and tyrosine (a precursor of thyroid hormones, catecholamines and melanin).[47]

Again, Elson Haas, M.D. writes, "Ascorbic acid was not **isolated** from lemons until 1932, though the scourge of scurvy, the vitamin C deficiency disease, had been present for thousands of years. Other cultures of the world discovered their own sources of vitamin C. Powdered rose hips, acerola cherries, or spruce needles were consumed regularly, usually as teas, to prevent the scurvy disease."[48] Today many vitamin C supplements feature rose hips or acerola on the label, but the consumer is misled into

---

46. Smolin, pages 300–301.

47. Merck, page 974.

48. Haas

believing that these foods are the main sources of vitamin C. In actuality, it is common for isolated vitamin C to be the **main ingredient** with only five or ten percent comprised of rose hips or acerola. Mixing whole foods in with isolated vitamins is unfortunately a common marketing ploy to fool consumers into thinking they are buying whole food supplements instead of isolated vitamins and minerals.

Vitamin C, chemically regarded as a weak acid, may become depleted in the presence of alkalis such as baking soda. It is also easily oxidized (destroyed by oxygen) and is sensitive to light and heat (including pasteurization). In the diet, vitamin C may be lost easily in cooking, exposure to air and heated water. Too much copper in water pipes or cooking pots may also diminish vitamin C content. Certain drugs may also deplete vitamin C levels.

Although we tend to think of oranges for vitamin C, because most orange juice is pasteurized (heated), only fresh-squeezed orange juice is a good source of vitamin C, not the store-bought kind.

Haas writes, "Vitamin C is a very complex and important vitamin." Yet, in defiance of this fact, "ascorbic acid" is a name that has become interchangeable with vitamin C despite that vitamin C, in its food state, is a complex containing **more than just ascorbic acid**.

The best-known sources of vitamin C are citrus fruits—oranges, lemons, limes, tangerines, and grapefruits. Also high in natural concentrations are acerola berries, rose hips, papayas, cantaloupes, and strawberries. Some plant and herb specialists, including author/researcher James Duke, Ph.D., claim that that there is no greater source of vitamin C than can be found in the rare Amazon rainforest berry known as *camu camu*. This unusual berry-like fruit contains more than twice the amount of vitamin C than found in the highest vitamin C foods of common use in the rest of the so-called "civilized" world. At 2.7 grams of ascorbic acid per 100 grams of fruit, the ascorbic acid content is nothing short of astounding![49]

49. "Natural food-Fruit Vitamin C Content": The Natural Food Hub, re: Romero, M.A,. Rodriguez, *et al* 'Determination of Vitamin C and Organic acids in various fruits by HPLC', *Journal of Chromatographic Science, Vol 30, Nov 1992, pages 433–437*

At this writing, however, it is difficult to obtain camu camu for supplementation, as the fruit is considerably difficult to store for transportation and subject to oxidation and mold. This is owing primarily to the intense humidity and heat of the rainforest where the plant must be harvested. The discovery of camu camu alone should be reason enough to protect our rainforests from eternal destruction.

Haas advises, "Good vegetable sources [of vitamin C] include red and green peppers (the best), broccoli, Brussels sprouts, tomatoes, asparagus, parsley, dark leafy greens, cabbage, and sauerkraut. There is not much available in the whole grains, seeds, and beans; however, when these are sprouted, their vitamin C content shoots up. Sprouts, then, are good foods for winter and early spring, when other fresh fruits and vegetables are not as available. Animal foods contain almost no vitamin C; though fish, if eaten raw, has enough to prevent deficiency symptoms."[50]

VITAMIN D

Like any other vitamin, vitamin D is never found alone in nature, and is a complex that works interdependently as "a member of a large and cooperative bone-making and bone-maintenance **team** made up of nutrients and other compounds."[51] Vitamin D is dependent upon vitamin A, vitamin C, the hormones parathormone and calcitonin, collagen, and minerals such as calcium, phosphorus, magnesium, and fluoride—composing the inorganic part of bone. Vitamin D is metabolized in the liver and then in the kidney where it is then considered to be the biologically functioning form of vitamin D. The major functions of vitamin D are to increase the efficiency of intestinal calcium absorption and to mobilize calcium stores from bone to maintain the serum calcium and phosphorus concentrations within the normal physiological range.

---

50. Haas

51. Whitney, page 253.

The richest food sources of vitamin D include fish oils, such as cod or halibut, and the flesh of oily fish such as sardines, salmon and mackerel, as well as some breads and cereal, mushrooms, and some egg yolks. Raw, grade A milk is also a good source of vitamin D. Recent evidence suggests that the vitamin D content in milk is variable, and 50 percent of milk samples tested did not contain at least 50 percent of what was stated on the label. Some milk samples do not contain *any* vitamin D. The results of such surveys may be attributable to the destruction of vitamin D due to pasteurization (which also destroys important enzyme activity in milk and dairy products). Most milk products therefore, are fortified with isolated vitamin D.

Biochemistry teaches that "milk is not a very good source of vitamin D, although its vitamin D content may be increased by irradiation [natural, not to be confused with food irradiation] with ultraviolet light. The vitamin D content of the body may be increased by exposure of the skin to ultraviolet rays from the sun, but care must be taken to avoid overexposure and consequent sunburn. For this reason, vitamin D is sometimes called 'the sunshine vitamin.'"[52]

Health columnist Gabe Mirkin, M.D. writes:

> We don't know exactly how much sunlight you need for good health, but a recent report from Turkey shows that women who wear veils have lower blood levels of vitamin D and therefore are at increased risk for suffering osteoporosis (*Journal of Women's Health & Gender-Based Medicine*, Volume 10, Issue 8, 2001).

> Food sources of vitamin D include egg yolks, liver, and fish oils from sardines, herring, salmon and other fatty fish. The vast majority of people on earth do not eat enough of these foods to meet their requirements for vitamin D, so they have to depend

---

[52.] Sackheim, page 429.

on sunlight. You get enough vitamin D to meet your requirements by exposing a few inches of skin to sunlight for less than
one half hour a day. Veiled women in Turkey rarely expose any
part of their bodies to sunlight, so they have low blood levels of
vitamin D that increase their risk for osteoporosis. Fortified milk
is not a particularly good source of vitamin D because the calcium uses up vitamin D, so you may need more than you get in
the milk to compensate.[53]

Vitamin D is well known for its ability to prevent rickets in children
and *osteomalacia* in adults. Sunshine seems to be the most important element in rickets prevention because of its unique role in the synthesis of
calciferol (vitamin D_2) in the skin. Calciferol is classified as a hormone, as
it is present in small amounts in the body, and may be present in adequate
quantities in natural foods. It is formed in the skin (far removed from tar-
get organs), its rate of synthesis (or dietary intake) requires careful control,
and its mechanism of action, like that of the estrogens, may be linked to
DNA-directed processes. "Another reason for considering calciferol as a
hormone is that it is closely linked with two other hormones, calcitonin
and the parathyroid hormone, in the control of the calcium level in the
blood."[54]

Rickets is characterized by improper mineralization during the development of the bones, resulting in soft bones. Restated, rickets is the result
of an inability to deposit calcium phosphate in the bones, causing them to
become soft and pliable, leading to deformity—wherein joints enlarge and
the ribs become beaded—referred to as *rachitic rosary*. Injections of small
amounts of calciferol or one of its derivatives, or adequate exposure to
sunlight, have prevented or cured rickets.

Osteomalacia is characterized by demineralization of previously formed
bone leading to increased softness and susceptibility to fracture. A diet low

---

[53.] Dr. Mirkin's E-Zine February 24, 2002

[54.] Sackheim, page 429.

in phosphorus and vitamin D may lead to osteomalacia, a rare condition suggesting that adults need less vitamin D than children do. Osteomalacia is more likely to occur in women after repeated pregnancies and periods of lactation during which there has been a deficiency of vitamin D. In adulthood, a lack of calcium and vitamin D may cause osteoporosis which, like osteomalacia, is characterized by decalcification and softening of the bones, but to a much greater extent.[55]

Vitamin D deficiency may result in muscle weakness, bony deformities, neuromuscular irritability causing muscle spasms of the larynx (laryngospasm) and hands (carpopedal spasm), generalized convulsions and tetany. Working to deposit calcium salts into bone and maintain calcium-phosphorus homeostasis, vitamin D is essential not only in the diet, but also, indirectly, from exposure to sunlight.

Vitamin D's Complexity

Vitamin D_1, originally called vitamin D, is actually a mixture of vitamins D_2 (ergocalciferol) and D_3 (cholecalciferol) which are co-constituents of the vitamin D complex stored in body fat. Both are referred to, generically speaking, as vitamin D. Vitamin D precursors produced in plants (especially yeast) and animals are converted to vitamin D by exposure to ultraviolet light. "There is mounting evidence that in the absence of any exposure to sunlight the RDA [recommended daily allowance] for vitamin D in adults is between 600 and 800 IU (20 µg/day)."[56]

A 1997 study out of Tufts University, Boston, showed that vitamin D levels in winter may lead to an increased risk of bone loss in elderly men

---

55. Sackheim, page 431.

56. American Society for Nutritional Sciences, 1999, re: Holick, M.F. (1994) Vitamin D - new horizons for the 21st century. *Am. J. Clin. Nutr.* 60:619–630; DeLuca, H.F. (1988) The vitamin D story: a collaborative effort of basic science and clinical medicine. FASEB J. 2:224–236.

and women. Results from this study, published in *The American Journal of Clinical Nutrition* showed that "vitamin D levels decrease in winter and parathyroid hormone levels increase. This may accelerate bone loss..."[57]

As with any isolated vitamin, excessive intake may lead to toxic states and symptomatology. Excessive quantities of vitamin D (more than 5,000-10,000 IU/day) have been linked to *hypercalcemia* (too much calcium in the bloodstream), *hypercalciuria* (excess calcium in the urine), kidney stones, and soft tissue calcifications.[58]

Vitamin D supplementation alone (as an isolate), although highly touted in its role in bone health, may not provide as much benefit as once predicted. The results of one recent study, reported in *Annals of Internal Medicine*, regarding the relationship between vitamin D intake and bone fractures in elderly people, has found that supplements did not reduce the incidence of fractures.[59]

VITAMIN E

Vitamin E is a complex of fat-soluble substances including eight naturally occurring compounds.[60] As a supplement vitamin E is at best incomplete, and like all other isolated substances, at worst it is a synthetic chemical compound. About 75 percent of the vitamin E found in food is the *gamma tocopherol* form, while supplements may not contain any gamma

---

[57.] *Vitamin News*, April /May 1997, re: *The Journal of Clinical Nutrition*, 1996

[58.] ibid.

[59.] *Vitamin Update*, July 1996, re: Annals of Internal Medicine, 124, 400–406.

[60.] American Society for Nutritional Sciences: Meydani, M. (1995) Vitamin E. *Lancet* 345: 170–175

Meydani, S.N., Wu, D., Santos, M.S. & Hayek, M.G. (1995) Antioxidants and immune response in aged persons: Overview of present evidence. Am. J. Clin. Nutr.; 62: 1463S-1462S ; Miller, R.D. & Hayes, K.C. (1982) Vitamin excess and toxicity. In: *Nutritional Toxicology* (Hathcock, J.N., ed.) vol. 1, pp. 81–133. Academic Press, New York, NY.

tocopherol. Taking very high doses of alpha tocopherol may displace gamma tocopherol.[61]

Vitamin E's most sought-after effect is as an antioxidant and is regarded as "the most effective chain-breaking lipid-soluble antioxidant in the biological membrane, where it contributes to membrane stability. It protects critical cellular structures against damage from oxygen free radicals and reactive products of lipid peroxidation."[62]

Vitamin E deficiency is most noted in reproductive failure, nutritional "muscular dystrophy," hemolytic anemia, and neurological and immunological abnormalities. Vitamin E is known to prevent sterility in animals, and some animals on a vitamin E-deficient diet have developed muscular dystrophy resulting in paralysis.[63]

Vitamin E deficiency may lead to shortened length of RBC [red blood cell] life. Newer studies have pointed to vitamin E's benefit to cardiac and skin tissues, although traditional medical literature claims that a vitamin E deficiency occurs rarely in humans, except in cases of premature infants with very low birth weight and patients who fail to absorb fat. With its combined antioxidant potential, including the ability to preserve vitamin A, and benefit to the heart and skin, vitamin E is considered an anti-aging nutrient. High serum vitamin E levels have been associated with reduced risk for coronary heart disease in men and women.[64]

Low vitamin E levels may be linked with angina (chest/heart pains) related to coronary artery spasm. Japanese researchers at Toyama University measured plasma vitamin E levels and total lipid levels in patients with various types of angina. The conclusion was that patients with "active variant angina" had vitamin E levels significantly lower than those seen in people

---

[61.] *Vitamin News* for April/May 1997

[62.] ibid

[63.] Sackheim, page 432.

[64.] ibid

with no evidence of coronary artery disease. "The researchers also found that vitamin E levels rose as patients remained free of angina attacks for six months or longer. Variant angina caused by coronary artery spasm can occur when a person is at rest, can happen at odd times of the day or night and is more common in women under the age of 50."[65]

Due to the synergists present in vitamin E-containing foods, some researchers argue that whole food sources may be effective where isolated vitamin E supplementation fails; as reported in *HealthNews*:

> Vitamin E's role in heart disease prevention continues to be a hot topic of debate. Last month, we told you about a British study that found a reduced risk of nonfatal heart attack in people who took large doses of vitamin E pills. Now a study in the May 2 *New England Journal of Medicine* finds that postmenopausal women who received the most **vitamin E from foods**—about 10 IU a day—were about 60 percent less likely to die of heart disease than those whose intake of the vitamin was lowest (about 5 IU). **Supplements appeared to have no effect.** Even without a definitive answer, it still makes sense to get at least the RDA (30 IU) of vitamin E from food. Good sources include seeds and nuts, vegetable oils, wheat germ, tuna fish, and oatmeal. [66]

As an antioxidant, vitamin E competes with air pollution to affect the health of skin tissue:

> Recent findings from a study reported at the annual meeting of the Oxygen Club of California suggest that the ozone found in air pollution may remove vitamin E from the uppermost layer of

---

65. *Circulation* 1996, 94.

66. Vitamin E from Foods May Reduce Women's Heart Disease Risk, *HealthNews* from the publishers of the *New England Journal of Medicine,* June 4, 1996; OnHealth, 2000 OnHealth Network Company

the skin. This can lead to an aggravation of skin problems such as eczema and psoriasis. Researchers at the University of California exposed the skin for two hours to ozone levels twice those of peak times for heavily smog-polluted regions. They then measured the vitamin E content of the skin and found a reduction of up to 25 percent. After a similar exposure for six consecutive days only about one quarter of the original vitamin E remained. Previous scientific studies have shown that skin problems worsen in highly polluted areas. The effect on vitamin E may offer an explanation. Vitamin E acts as an antioxidant and protects against free radical damage. Loss of vitamin E may lead to the breakdown of fat molecules which regulate the movement of substances in and out of the skin. This breakdown may also trigger inflammatory responses in the lower layers of the skin.[67]

As time goes by, studies continue to elucidate vitamin E's role in biochemistry, showing that this vitamin complex provides a multitude of health benefits affecting behavior, menopausal symptoms, hormonal balance, skin health, cardiovascular function, cellular protection, intellect and brain function.

Austrian researchers assessed vitamin E levels and intellectual function in nearly 1,800 adults aged from 50 to 75 to discover that the vitamin may prevent age-related decline in brain function. Reported in the *Journal of the American Geriatrics Society,* 1998, the study showed that those with higher vitamin E levels were less likely to have low scores on tests of intellectual capacity. Such tests are used to assess decline in Alzheimer's disease and other types of dementia.[68]

[67.] *Vitamin News* for April/May 1997

[68.] *Journal of the American Geriatrics Society* 1998;46:1407–10: from *Vitamin News* March 1999.

Vitamin E Food Factors & Selenium

There are many studies performed on the efficacy of isolated vitamin E supplementation against disease, but scant research exists on vitamin E-containing foods wherein the vitamin E complex coexists with its natural cofactors. However, although few in number, the latter studies indicate that vitamin E-containing foods lower the risk of disease. At this writing, researchers can only speculate that it is the entire combination of vitamins, minerals and other dietary (as opposed to supplemental) nutrients that take credit for any salubrious results. For instance, a long-term Nurses Health Study beginning in 1976 proclaimed that eating nuts reduces heart disease risk. This study suggests that women who frequently include nuts in their diet have a reduced risk of coronary heart disease. Involving more than 80,000 women aged from 34 to 59 who had not been diagnosed with any kind of heart disease, researchers collected detailed information on the medical histories and lifestyles of nurses. Every two years, the women receive a follow-up questionnaire. During the 14-year follow-up period for this part of the study, there were 861 cases of non-fatal heart attack and 394 cases of fatal coronary heart disease. Analysis of the results showed that women who ate more than five ounces (approximately 150g) of nuts per week had a 35 percent lower risk of coronary heart disease than women who ate no nuts or ate less than 1 ounce (approximately 30g) per month.

Results from the Physicians Health Study, reported at the annual meeting of the American Heart Association, also suggest that eating nuts can reduce the risk of death from heart attack. The results of this study, which lasted for 11 years and involved more than 22,000 male doctors, show that "the risk of total and sudden heart attack decreased with increasing nut consumption."[69] Nuts contain a wide array of nutrients and are known to have beneficial effects on blood fats, decreasing total cholesterol and LDL cholesterol levels. The study proclaimed that the benefits of eating nuts was

---

[69]. *British Medical Journal* 1998;317:1341–45 ; from *Vitamin News* 70. March 1999.

owing to their potentially protective compounds, which include not only vitamin E, but also magnesium, selenium, protein, fiber, potassium and alpha linolenic acid. The results of this study support the efficacy of vitamin E as a nutrient component of whole food, with its complement of synergistic nutrients intact.

As with many other nutrients, vitamin E deficiency may occur secondarily (not necessarily due to inadequate dietary intake), by way of digestive difficulties, e.g., malabsorption syndrome, as in cases of sprue, celiac disease, cystic fibrosis or biliary atresia (congenital absence or closure of a normal body orifice or tubular organ).[70]

Food Sources of Vitamin E & Selenium

Food sources of vitamin E, in its entire, naturally occurring complex, include wheat germ and wheat germ oil, as well as in the oils of most grains and seeds (including sunflower). Other sources include milk, eggs, fish, muscle meats, cereals, leafy vegetables and oils such as cottonseed, corn, palm and peanut. J.E. Meyers Botanical Gardens of Hammond, Indiana, reports that watercress is one of the best sources of vitamin E. Dried watercress may contain triple the amount of vitamin E found in dried lettuce leaves.[71] The value of vitamin E in any food, however, must be considered in the raw state, as this vitamin is subject to oxidation and destruction in the presence of ultraviolet light, refining, extreme heating and processing.

One of the most important cofactors in vitamin E foods (not found in vitamin E supplements within the food complex) is selenium, a celebrated antioxidant mineral. Herbalist James Duke, Ph.D. states that the average Brazil nut (a vitamin E food) contains the daily value (recommended daily intake) for selenium (70mg).[72]

---

[70]. Merck, page 966.

[71]. Hutchens, Alma R., *Indian Herbology of North America*, Shambhala, Boston, 1991, page 293.

[72]. Duke, *The Green Pharmacy*, page 24.

The importance of vitamin E foods is understated in light of today's processed diet and exposure to environmental toxins. The many antioxidant, cancer and cardiovascular studies underway show great interest in the protective value of not only vitamin E, but also of the foods wherein this vitamin is contained because of the existing synergists. As part of the vitamin E complex, essential fatty acids (as well as selenium) are important cofactors not to be overlooked. "The major symptom of vitamin E deficiency in humans is an increase in red blood cell fragility. Since vitamin E is absorbed from the intestines in chylomicrons [mainly triglyceride fat particles], any fat malabsorption diseases can lead to deficiencies in vitamin E intake. Neurological disorders have been associated with vitamin E deficiencies associated with fat malabsorptive disorders. Increased intake of vitamin E is recommended in premature infants fed formulas that are low in the vitamin as well as in persons consuming a diet high in polyunsaturated fatty acids. Polyunsaturated fatty acids tend to form free radicals upon exposure to oxygen, and this may lead to an increased risk of certain cancers."[73]

Regarding the vitamin E co-nutrient selenium, the American Society for Nutritional Sciences reports:

Selenium (Se) is an essential trace element that functions as a component of enzymes involved in antioxidant protection and thyroid hormone metabolism…Selenium deprivation reduces activities of the selenium-dependent [enzymes] peroxidases and deiodinases. The signs in animals depend upon vitamin E status and appear only when both nutrients are limiting. They vary according to species. For example, selenium-and vitamin E-deficient animals show myopathies of skeletal (e.g., sheep, cow, horse), cardiac (pig) or smooth (dog, cow) muscle; hepatic necrosis (rat, pig); increased capillary permeability (chicken); or pancreatic acinar

---

73. King

degeneration (chicken). Characteristic signs of selenium deficiency have not been described in humans, but very low selenium status is a factor in the etiologies of a juvenile cardiomyopathy (Keshan Disease) and a chondrodystrophy [abnormal development of cartilage] (Kaschin-Beck Disease) that occur in selenium-deficient regions of China.[74]

Important sources of selenium are mostly in "vitamin E foods": meats, fish and grains. As stated, of particular note are Brazil nuts, known to have relatively high selenium concentrations. Recent research on selenium points to its anti-tumorigenic effects, yet, "The mechanism(s) of anti-tumorigenic effects of selenium and the possible role of selenium in affecting the risk of human cancer are not clear."[75]

---

[74]. American Society for Nutritional Sciences, 1999, re: Burk, R.F., ed. (1994) Selenium in Biology and Human Health. Springer-Verlag, New York, NY; Combs, G.F., Jr. (1994) Essentiality and toxicity of selenium: a critique of the Recommended Dietary Allowances and the Reference Dose. In: Risk Assessment of Essential Elements (Mertz, C., Abernathy, C. & Olin, S.S., eds.), pp. 167–183. International Life Sciences Institute Press, Washington, DC.

[75]. ibid

OTHER NUTRIENTS FOUND IN NATURE'S FOOD COMPLEXES

There are many other substances found in Nature's whole foods of benefit to our bodies. These ingredients make up parts of the whole food "complex" and are rarely found in supplement form (except whole food concentrate supplements), especially not in vitamin, mineral or multivitamin pills. Many of these food substances are called *phytochemicals* or *phytonutrients*, meaning that they are plant-based nutrients, but are generally not recognized as widely as vitamins, minerals and proteins. Other substances may only be referred to as "micronutrients," but in spite of this uninspiring term, should never be considered less than important in the larger scheme of the study of nutrition.

To overlook the value of micronutrients and their ability to promote life and vitality is to ignore the splendor of the food complex as the essence of nutrition. The larger nutrients (macronutrients) such as vitamins, carbohydrates, minerals, and the rest, though receiving the most attention, have no value without the underlying support of micronutrients such as trace minerals. Further, all of these elements in the food complex must exist within a delicate, natural balance for the optimum promotion of health and healing. David Yarrow, author of New York state's first organic certification standards, explains:

> It's important to realize that in dealing with minerals, whether in the human bloodstream or the soil, it's the proportions that are important. If we load up the soil with one mineral, it makes the other minerals seem to be deficient in relation to the oversupply of that one mineral...One other feature of this situation is that

trace elements have a tremendous amount of power. They may be the "least" of the elements, but because of their critical functions in creating enzymes and hormones and their role in immune and reproduction functions in plants, the loss of a small amount of a trace element is much more dramatic to the health of a plant than the loss of a large amount of a primary mineral. The power of the trace elements is amplified by the biological uses that they are put to.[76]

In this chapter we will briefly look at SOME of the substances found in nature's foods, but this is by no means a complete or extensive list, nor is it in any particular order, for how can we justifiably claim that one nutrient is more important than another if, without one, deficiency and disease surely follows? The intention here is to make us think about the importance of whole, natural foods by virtue of their complexities, with respect for and recognition of all substances large and small.

Pigments

Plant pigments are often spoken of as part of the whole food complex, yet these colorful components are rarely defined in terms of their value. To many species of animals and insects, the colors of plants make them attractive and recognizable for consumption. Plant color also provides camouflage from natural predators, and we know that certain colors attract and absorb the sun's rays to different degrees. Pigments also absorb energy and offer this energy to us when we eat the plant, making many pigmented plants (containing chlorophyll, carotenes, etc.) health-promoting foods.

The orange pigment, beta carotene—best known of the plant color compounds—first caught researchers' eyes when population studies linked low rates of certain cancers with a high intake

---

76. *Acres, USA*, "Earth Restoration: Nuturing Soil & Trees to Heal Our Planet, interview with David Yarrow, February 2002, page 26

of fruits and vegetables containing lots of beta carotene. A current theory holds that cancer, heart disease, stroke, and other diseases of aging result from cumulative damage to cells by free radicals—most of which our cells generate through ordinary metabolism. So nutrition and medical researchers are dissecting the fruits and vegetables consumed by healthy populations, looking for the best combinations to prevent such damage. What they are finding is that **fruits and vegetables contain hundreds of other pigments besides beta carotene**—as well as non-pigment compounds—that may play a role in preventing oxidative damage. [These other pigments are absent in isolated vitamin A and beta carotene supplements].

Studies to date suggest many pigmented plant chemicals, [phytochemicals], appear to maintain health by boosting the immune system, reducing inflammation and allergies, detoxifying contaminants and pollutants, and/or activating enzymes that block unbridled cell division. Fred Khachik, a chemist with ARS [Agricultural Research Service], points out that the diets of most people supply more of two other carotenoids—lutein and lycopene—than they do beta carotene.[77]

Enzymes

Enzymes are very special substances made up of the proteins responsible for speeding up and enabling biochemical processes. In the simplest of terms, we can say that enzymes "make things happen." They are like keys that unlock doors to cellular functions. Without enzymes, there would be no life on earth. On a more personal note, without enzymes there would

---

[77.] McBride, Judy, *Agricultural Research/*, November 1996, ARS; Jean Mayer USDA Human Nutrition Research Center on Aging, Tufts University, Boston, MA

be no life in us; none of our cells could function. There are countless numbers of enzymes with all sorts of functions. Some help digest foods while others help get rid of waste, some manufacture blood cells and others dissolve blood clots, some speed up healing and others stimulate the immune system; and so on. Enzymes must come from the foods we eat or we suffer the fate of premature aging, illness and systemic malfunctioning. If we eat dead, processed, refined foods, then we are not eating naturally, and we are not consuming needed enzymes. When we eat a dead diet of foul nutrition, we put a tremendous burden on our bodies, using our own bodily enzymes to try to digest food particles made of fats, amino acids and carbohydrates.

Certainly, vitamin pills do not provide us with enzymes. As a result of eating the modern diet lacking in enzymes, digestive difficulties have become the norm. These difficulties include gas, bloating, mucous buildup, high cholesterol, stomach/intestinal cramping, heartburn and more—the very reason why Dad has to slump back in his chair and unbutton his trousers even in front of the dinner guests or in the fanciest restaurant in town! When foods are not digested, their nutrients are not made available to us, resulting in more serious, long-term and chronic illnesses, including diseases of the circulatory, cardiovascular, respiratory, gastrointestinal/ digestive, lymphatic and musculoskeletal systems, to name a few.

Enzymes are components of real, whole foods and living organisms. Enzymes are used to enable and speed up chemical reactions, such as breaking down food into smaller particles for digestion and causing blood to clot. Each enzyme carries on a very specific function within cells. Many researchers say, as we age we continue to diminish our supply of enzymes and enable the onset of disease and aging. We need enzymes in our foods to help slow down the aging process, to keep our cells protected with immune functions and to allow cellular activities, such as the production of energy and the removal of wastes, to take place .

The topic of enzymes is best explained by Dr. Edward Howell, one of the modern pioneers in enzyme study:

> There are three classes of enzymes: metabolic enzymes, which run our bodies; digestive enzymes, which digest our food; and food enzymes from raw foods, which start food digestion. Our bodies—all our organs and tissues—are run by metabolic enzymes. These enzyme workers take proteins, fats, and carbohydrates (starches, sugars, etc.), and structure them into healthy bodies, keeping everything working properly. Every organ and tissue has its own particular metabolic enzymes to do specialized work. One authority made an investigation and found 98 distinct enzymes working in the arteries, each with a a particular job to do. The liver has numerous different enzymes working. No one has ever investigated how many specific enzymes are needed to run the heart, brain, lungs, kidneys, etc.
>
> Since good health depends on all of these metabolic enzymes doing an excellent job, we must be sure that nothing interferes with the body making enough of them. A shortage could mean trouble, many times serious. Modern research is implicating enzymes in all of our activities. Even thinking involves some enzyme activity…Hundreds of metabolic enzymes are necessary to carry on the work of the body—to repair damage and decay.[78]

According to Howell, there is a relationship between the enzymes we use for digestion and those we use for metabolic processes. Howell explains that we have an "enzyme potential" that limits the amount of enzymes our bodies produce over the course of our lives. If we do not eat enough enzyme-containing foods, we more rapidly use up our inherent

---

[78.] Howell, Edward, *Enzyme Nutrition: The Food Enzyme Concept*, Avery Publishing Group, New Jersey, 1985, page 3

enzyme potential. He writes that if our foods do not contain enzymes, then we are burdening our bodies by using up valuable metabolic enzymes, because "there is competition between the two classes of enzymes...

"If humans take in more exogenous (outside) digestive enzymes, as nature ordained, the enzyme potential will not have to waste so much of its heritage digesting food. It can distribute more of this precious commodity to the metabolic enzymes, where it rightfully belongs. This rightful distribution of enzyme energy will not only act to maintain health and prevent disease, but is expected to help cure established disease. The old saying that nature will cure really refers to metabolic enzyme activity, because there is no other mechanism in the body to cure anything."[79]

Enzymes should not be underestimated in their importance to life and health, but unfortunately, processed, overcooked, refined and packaged foods—and this represents the bulk of the American diet—do not contain enzymes. If one were to have for dinner a bowl of hot soup followed by a baked potato, a barbecued steak and a side order of cooked green beans, such a meal would contain zero enzymes. As you can see, this is not a rare example of a modern evening meal.

Vitamin and multivitamin supplements do not contain food enzymes.

As we age, we need enzymes more than ever. One leading expert tells us, "This is when enzymes from fresh fruits and vegetables, food concentrates, and supplements from animal, microbial and plant sources can help."[80]

Some of the most important enzymes studied in the field of nutrition are those that break down fats (lipase), carbohydrates (amylase, ptyalin, pancreatin), and proteins (protease, hydrochloric acid, bromelain, rennin, papain, trypsin), fiber (cellulase) and sugars (maltase, sucrase, etc.). Primarily these enzymes receive a lot of attention because of their role in

---

[79.] ibid, page 5

[80.] Cichoke, p. 1

enabling digestion; yet we cannot forget the life-supporting importance of the millions of other enzymes inherent in Nature's foods.

Coenzymes

Coenzymes are enzymes that work with other enzymes. They are nonprotein, and they form active enzymes when combined with specific proteins. Many times, coenzymes are regarded as vitamins and are best described as enzyme helpers. Our bodies do not manufacture coenzymes; they come from our food, food supplements and enzyme supplements. Recent scientific discoveries have begun to shed light on the value of coenzymes, with much emphasis placed on coenzyme Q10 for heart health, to be discussed in a subsequent chapter.

Chlorophyll

Now here's a substance you'll never find in your bottle of vitamins and minerals! Many of our "green foods" are the source of important vitamin A precursors, vitamin C, minerals such as zinc, phosphorus, iron and calcium, and trace elements. Such substances, when removed from (or isolated from) the green food to be made in to a supplement, leave behind the very valuable chlorophyll component. Researchers are only just beginning to understand the value of chlorophyll as a healing agent, both topically and internally.

Dorland's Medical Dictionary defines chlorophyll as the green coloring matter of plants by which photosynthesis is accomplished. There are many types, including, but not limited to, bluish green chlorophyll found in oxygen-releasing plants; a yellowish-green chlorophyll; chlorophyll found in marine algae; a red variety occurring in red algae; and bacteriochlorophylls found in phototropic bacteria. Water-soluble chlorophyll derivatives, "consisting mainly of the copper complex of the sodium and/or potassium salts of chlorophyll, are applied topically to the skin for deodorization, for enhancement of normal tissue repair, and for relief of itching in various skin lesions. Preparations of the derivatives for oral administration are used to deodorize certain necrotic, ulcerative lesions, to control fecal and urinary odors in colostomy, ileostomy or incontinence, and to deodorize urinary and fecal fistulas and breath and body odors not related to faulty hygiene."[81]

Chlorophyll is a lipid—a macromolecule (large molecule) of the oily or waxy class that is insoluble in water but soluble in oil, forming biologically important pigments. Plants and other photosynthetic organisms use chlorophyll to absorb light with great efficiency. In a complex system, the **captured light is converted into energy.**

Good dietary sources of chlorophyll include plant foods with dark green leaves such as spinach, kale, lettuce and parsley. Within the last 20 years or so, chlorella, wheat grass, barley grass and algae (including spirulina) have gained added attention for their chlorophyll content. Although many promises and anecdotal accounts tell of chlorophyll's miraculous role in healing, scant scientific literature exists on chlorophyll's curative abilities. However, some preliminary evidence suggests that chlorophyll might be helpful in detoxifying cancer-promoting substances.[82]

In natural health care, chlorophyll is recommended in nutritional schedules in perles or whole, green food concentrated supplements for hormonal support, detoxification, blood platelet health and in the healing of internal and external wounds. Author Ronald Seibold, MS writes,

> The action of chlorophyll on wounds has a unique feature. Most medicines become less effective with repeated use. In contrast,

---

[81]. Dorland's. p. 211.

[82]. Lininger, page 281; re: Gruskin B. Chlorophyll — its therapeutic place in acute and suppurative disease. *American Journal of Surgery* 1940; 49–56; Ayatsu H, Negishi T, Arimoto S, et. al. Porphyrins as potential inhibitors against exposure to carcinogens and mutagens. *Mutat Res* 1993: 290; 79–85.

an initial application of chlorophyll makes a wound more sensitive to its healing benefits with repeated use...{Researcher} Dr. G.H. Collings considered chlorophyll to "have the most constant and marked effect of all agents for stimulating cell proliferation and tissue repair." Collings demonstrated that the healing time of wounds is shorter with chlorophyll therapy than with penicillin, vitamin D, sulfanilamide or no treatment.

Chlorophyll also accelerates wound healing by reducing hemagglutination [the clumping together of erythrocytes that may be caused by antibodies, viruses or substances such as high-molecular weight dextrans] and inflammation. When a tissue is injured, foreign substances in the blood generally cause blood cells to clump together. This limits the amount of nutrients available for repair of the injured tissue. When chlorophyll is administered to a wound, this clumping is reduced, so the lag time associated with tissue repair is shortened. Chlorophyll decreases swelling by reducing the synthesis of fibrin (the protein associated with blood clot formation). This gives chlorophyll a mild blood thinning, or heparin-like property, which can enhance the effectiveness of local immune defenses.

Chlorophyll has also been shown to be extremely effective in speeding the healing of peptic ulcers, wounds which develop internally in the gastrointestinal tract. Several studies document the use of chlorophyll in the treatment of ulcers resistant to more conventional therapies...In the Offenkrantz study, 20 of the 27 patients with chronic ulcers were relieved of pain and other symptoms in 24 to 27 hours. Complete healing of the damaged tissues, as demonstrated by x-ray examination, occurred in 20 of 24 cases within two to seven weeks. These reports include case descriptions of dramatic recoveries from severe, long standing problems...

European investigators report preliminary favorable results in the use of chlorophyll in the treatment of pancreatitis. The chlorophyll is thought to influence several enzymatic reactions which complicate this disease.[83]

Carotenes, Carotenoids

Carotenes harvest light for a plant that can be converted into energy and used in the production of chlorophyll. Carotenes act as protective agents instrumental in preventing chlorophyll from being damaged by oxygen.

As discussed under the heading "Vitamin A," carotenes are substances that are converted from foods by the body (in the liver) to vitamin A. As such, these are very important nutrients, given the importance of vitamin A to our cells.

Although beta carotene is now a popular as a supplement, the fact remains that there are more than 500 other carotenoids found in the plant kingdom. Carotenoids are efficient at absorbing light that is used for energy within plants and animals; carotenoids are the major yellow and red pigments in many fruits and vegetables. Beta-carotene and alpha-carotene are responsible for the orange color of carrots, and lycopene for

---

[83.] Seibold, page 45–47, citing: Smith, L 1955. The present status of topical chlorophyll therapy. *The NY State Journal of Medicine*, March, 1940; Chernomorsky, S and Segelman, A, 1988; Biological activities of chlorophyll derivatives, *New Jersey Medicine*, 85:669–673; Young, R and Beregi, J, 1980, Use of chlorophyllin in the care of geriatric patients, *Journal of the American geriatrics Society*, 28:46–47, 1980; Miller, J, Jackson, D and Collier, C, 1960. The inhibition of Russell's viper venom by the water-soluble derivatives of sodium-copper chlorophyllin. *American Journal of Surgery*, 99:48–49; Miller, J, Jackson, D and Collier, C, 1958, The inhibition of clotting by chlorophyllin, *American Journal of Surgery*, 95: 967–969; Sack, P and Barnard, R, 1955, Studies on the hemagglutinating and inflammation properties of exudate from nonhealing wounds and their inhibition by chlorophyll derivatives. *New York State Journal of Medicine*, October 15, 1955, p. 2952–2956.

the red color of tomatoes; astaxanthin imparts a red or pink color to lobsters and salmon. Biochemically speaking, the term "carotene" refers to
carotenoids containing only carbon and hydrogen (e.g. beta-carotene,
alpha-carotene, lycopene), while the term "xanthophylls" refers to compounds containing hydroxyl groups (lutein, zeaxanthin, beta-cryptoxanthin) or keto groups (canthaxanthin) or both (astaxanthin).

Although many studies indicate that a diet rich in fruits and vegetables
seems to protect against cancer and heart attacks (among other diseases),
with beta carotene as well as other nutrient complexes (including antioxidants) providing the protection, evidence indicates that isolated beta
carotene supplementation fails to offer what whole food complexes provide. In simpler terms, we need more than just beta-carotene to be healthy
and cure disease. Despite the popularity of beta carotene supplements, the
New England Journal of Medicine reported the results of a study on beta
carotene **supplements** only to reveal their lack of effect on the incidence of
cancer and heart disease:

> There have been a small number of studies which have found
> beta carotene to have no protective effect, but it was felt that a
> larger study over a longer period of time was necessary to fully
> investigate the disease prevention possibilities. The Physicians
> Health Study in the United States is one such major project. In
> this study 22,000 male doctors were given 50 mg of beta carotene
> or placebo every other day for an average of 12 years. The study
> found that the beta carotene supplements produced neither ben-
> efit nor harm in the doctors that were taking them as they did not
> significantly protect against heart disease or cancer.[84]

The key discovery here is—as earnest researchers have been trying to
shout out above the noise of marketing hype—that there is much more to
the body's nutrient requirements than can be addressed by isolated substances

---

[84.] *New England Journal of Medicine*, Volume 334, No 18.

(vitamin A or beta-carotene supplements) alone. There is no question that beta carotene is a health-promoting part of foods, yet in various instances it is of questionable value (and possibly harmful) as an isolated supplement.

A 1998 study from Sweden of 124 men and women with lung cancer and 235 people without the disease measured the benefit of a fruit-and-vegetable diet. Findings showed that the risk of lung cancer was 30 percent lower in those who ate a great amount of vegetables, and 40 percent lower in those consuming "a lot of non-citrus fruits." Results of the study showed that carrots reduced the risk of lung cancer. Researchers speculate that the high beta carotene content in these foods may be the key to lung cancer prevention.[85]

Another Swedish study also reported on the benefits of foods (not isolated supplements) containing beta carotene with similar optimistic results. The findings were that high beta carotene diets lower breast cancer risk. Of 644 women in this study, 273 had been diagnosed with breast cancer. The women were asked to recall details about their diets throughout their lives. Those reporting diets rich in beta carotene foods for 20 years or more were found to be in the lower risk category than women whose diets included beta carotene only in more recent years, or whose diets were traditionally low in beta carotene foods.[86]

Diets high in beta carotene-containing fruits and vegetables, under study by a team of Dutch researchers in the late 1990s, show a correlation with reduced risk of heart attack. As part of a four-year Rotterdam study, researchers followed the dietary and medical histories of 4,802 people aged from 55 to 95. Out of 124 of the participants who had heart attacks during this period, analysis showed that those with the highest daily intakes of beta carotene had a 45 percent lower risk of heart attack, compared to people consuming the lowest amount of beta carotene.[87]

---

[85]. *International Journal of Cancer* 1998;78:430–6.

[86]. *Epidemiology* 1999;10:49–53

[87]. *American Journal of Clinical Nutrition* 1999; 69:261–6.

Lycopene & Tomatoes

As another component of the vitamin A carotenoid complex, **lycopene** has also been studied in its original food form. Lycopene is the carotenoid which gives tomatoes their red color and is one of the major carotenoids in the diet of North Americans and Europeans. It is found in high concentration in the testes, adrenal gland and prostate. Levels of lycopene seem to decrease with age. Several studies suggest that dietary lycopene may help prevent cardiovascular disease and cancers of the prostate, pancreas and gastrointestinal tract. According to the results of a 1997 study conducted in Germany, lycopene from tomato paste is more bio-available (easy for our bodies to use) than lycopene from fresh tomatoes. In a study published in 1995, researchers at Harvard Medical School assessed the links between diet during a one-year period and prostate cancer in almost 48,000 men taking part in the Health Professionals Follow-up Study. They found that men who ate more foods high in lycopene, such as tomatoes, pizza and tomato sauce, were less likely to be at risk of prostate cancer.[88]

Other Carotenoid Health Benefits

In consideration of the carotenoid complex, data from the Third National Health and Nutrition Examination Survey suggest prevention against diabetes is also a benefit of diets full of vitamin A foods. "Researchers from the Centers for Disease Control and Prevention in Atlanta, Georgia, examined concentrations of alpha carotene, beta carotene, cryptoxanthin, lutein/zeaxanthin, and lycopene in 1,010 people (aged from 40 to 74) with normal glucose tolerance [the body's ability to manage sugars normally]. These were compared with those from 277 people with impaired glucose tolerance and 148 people with newly diagnosed diabetes. The results showed that beta carotene and lycopene concentrations were highest in those with normal glucose tolerance, lower in those with impaired

---

[88]. Reavley, 1999, re: *Journal of the National Cancer Institute* 1999; 91: 317–331

glucose tolerance and even lower in people with newly diagnosed diabetes." These results add weight to the evidence that nutrients in fruit and vegetables reduce the risk of developing diabetes.[89]

Carotenes are found in carrots, yams, cantaloupe, dandelion, wheat grass, squash and many other green and yellow vegetables; and are presumed to enhance the body's immune system by acting as antioxidants and feeding the liver the building blocks of vitamin A.

Although *beta* carotene is a popular ingredient in supplements, as noted, it is only one of 600 substances found in whole foods under the category of carotenoids; so when you consume beta-carotene supplements, you are leaving out the rest of the carotenoids. A variety of raw, whole foods, of course, carries the array of carotenoids needed for various cellular functions.

Flavonoids, Bioflavonoids, Vitamin F

Flavonoids are sometimes called vitamin F. Also called *bioflavonoids*, these nutrients are plant-based, especially occurring in fruits and berries. Flavonoids include flavones (subunits) such as anthocyanin, catechin, tannin, quercitin and other hard-to-pronounce substances that carry on specific functions that include antioxidant tasks. (Antioxidants are substances in foods that keep cells from being damaged by oxygen-robbing molecules such as drugs, chemicals and pollutants). By the 1950s scientists recognized that flavonoids work together with vitamin C in foods, especially to support and heal blood vessels and to control bleeding. In fact, easy bruising is often a symptom of the need for flavonoid foods. Recent research continues to show the importance of flavonoids, especially in eye health (to prevent and combat glaucoma and macular degeneration), cardiovascular health, inflammation and health of the skin, gums and soft tissue.

---

[89]. Reavley, 1999, re: American Journal of Epidemiology 1999; 149: 168–76

More than 5,000 flavonoids have been identified, with at least more than 60 in citrus fruits alone. Anthocyanins, a subgroup of flavonoids, accounts for the majority of yellow, red and blue pigmentation in foods. Another subgroup, formerly referred to as vitamin P, is called *bioflavonoids*, and includes citrin, rutin, hesperidin, quercitin, myricetin and kampferol, and others (the latter three are known to help prevent cataracts and protect foods from oxidation). Certain other bioflavonoids such as nobiletin and tangerin, can stimulate enzymes that detoxify our bodies from drugs and carcinogenic chemicals.[90]

Bioflavonoids are regarded as substances in foods concerned with the maintenance of a normal state of walls of small blood vessels. *Dorlands Medical Dictionary* explains, "Flavonoids are grouped in order of increasing oxidation state: catechins; leucoanthocyanidins and flavanones, flavanols, flavones, and anthocyanidins; and flavonols."[91]

Acting as antioxidants (substances that keep oxygen from destroying other substances at the cellular level), flavonoids guard against the oxygen-robbing effects of free radicals (substances that "steal" oxygen from healthy cells) that are present in environmental pollutants as well as within the human body (generated as a result of metabolic functions). "Flavonoids can stabilize connective tissue and capillaries, and seem to work together with vitamin C in this regard. They also decrease [actually aid the process of] inflammation by several mechanisms."[92] Flavonoids block enzymes that cause difficulties with inflammation, and they desensitize mast cells (a type of immune cell embedded in tissues that release inflammatory agents like histamine when they encounter a foreign invader). Various flavonoids decrease the ability of platelets to form dangerous blood clots. Flavonoids

---

[90.] Reuben, C.A., Carolyn and Joan Priestley, M.D., *Essential Supplements for Women*, Perigee Books, New York, 1988, page 88.

[91.] *Dorlands Illustrated Medical Dictionary*, 26th Edition, W.B. Saunders, Philadelphia,1985, page 509.

[92.] Ronzio, page 350.

can either activate or inhibit detoxification enzymes of the liver that help dispose of wastes and toxic materials.

Flavonoids help stimulate the production of collagen, a fibrous protein that forms connective tissue that holds cells together.

"Very likely, combinations of flavonoids together with other factors in foods will be most beneficial. The long term effects of purified flavonoids [isolated substances] on health have not been fully investigated. It should be pointed out that certain flavonoids can actually increase oxidation (pro-oxidant effects) and that high levels could inhibit the thyroid gland."[93]

Recent scientific studies have shown that certain bioflavonoids, such as those in the fruit called bilberry, have decreased the damage to eyes and reduced the diseases known as macular degeneration and glaucoma. Bioflavonoids are also instrumental in keeping blood vessels strong in the extremities, such as those in the legs that cause so-called spider veins. Further, bioflavonoids reduce the incidences of easy bruising as well as the healing of bruises.

Bioflavonoids coexist alongside vitamins and minerals but are not contained in their natural state in vitamin or multivitamin pills.

One recent study shows that high intakes of flavonoids reduce the risk of heart attack by as much as one third, according to researchers at the University of Minnesota in Minneapolis. "The researchers examined the links between heart attack and stroke and intake of three major sources of flavonoids—apples, broccoli and tea. The results showed a 38 per cent reduction in heart disease deaths among women with the highest levels of flavonoid intake compared to those with the lowest daily intake."[94]

[93.] Ronzio, p. 181

[94.] Vitamin News, online October 1999, re: American Journal of Epidemiology 1999;149:943–949

Xanthophylls

Xanthophylls are one of any of several yellow accessory pigments found in plant leaves, egg yolks and human blood plasma. These pigments come from carotenes and are involved in photosynthesis—the capture of energy. Xanthophylls are not converted by our bodies into vitamin A.

Terpenes

Terpenes are another form of phytochemical (plant ingredient), and are found in citrus fruit, caraway seeds, licorice root and other fruits and vegetables. Terpenes are chiefly contained in essential oils, resins and other vegetable aromatic products. With subgroups of monoterpenes and triterpenes, terpenes are being studied for their promise in blocking the action of carcinogens (cancer-causing agents) and inhibiting hormone-related cancers.[95]

Terpenes are long-chain lipids (fatty substances) of great biochemical importance and include chlorophyll as well as the pigment retinal which absorbs light in the eyes.[96] Many terpenes are important plant defensive compounds. For example, the smell of pine trees and the sticky sap that pine trees give off are largely mixtures of terpenes. Terpenes build and create steroids as well.

Antioxidants

One of the biggest problems we face with pollution and chemicals is the destruction of our cells as these chemicals are robbers of healthy molecules

---

[95]. Ronzio, page 350.

[96]. Raven, Peter H., Director, Missouri Botanical Garden; Engelmann Professor of Botany, Washington University, St. Louis, Missouri and George B Johnson, Professor of Biology, Washington University, St. Louis, Missouri : *Biology*, Third Edition Mosby-Year Book, Inc., Missouri, 1992, pages 49–50.

of oxygen. Antioxidants are not specific food nutrients, but they exist as part of the food complex—a function of certain food constituents. There are many kinds of antioxidants; some are vitamins, some are bioflavonoids, and some are other substances (such as the mineral selenium). Antioxidants, as natural food particles, protect our cells from damage due to "free radicals" (oxygen robbers). Antioxidants are found in a wide variety of foods, ranging from green vegetables to wheat germ, and from seeds and nuts to pure drinking water. There are many nutrients that possess antioxidant properties that not only protect our bodies from harm, but also protect vitamins and other nutrients from destruction. Scientists are currently studying the effects of antioxidants against major illnesses such as cancer, arthritis and so-called auto-immune diseases.

Phytoestrols, Phytosterols, Phytoestrogens

Robert Ronzio, Ph.D., author of *The Encyclopedia of Nutrition & Good Health*, defines phytoestrols as plant-based substances which mimic the influences of the female sex hormone estrogen. Thus, it is believed that phytoestrols (also called phytoestrogens) may inhibit some cancers, including breast cancer. Whole foods such as soybeans, lentils, various legumes and peas are sources of phytoestrogens. Phytoestrogens are believed to support estrogen functions in the body. Estrogens cause cells in certain parts of the body to proliferate—to increase in number. They promote the cellular health of the vagina, uterus, pelvis, breasts and fatty tissues deposited in areas such as the thighs and hips. (Phytoestrogens occurring naturally in whole foods are not harmful for males to ingest). By the way, synthetic ("man-made") estrogen, administered to regulate hormonal dysfunction, has been reported to cause serious health problems, including cancer in females.

Plant estrogens, states nutritional researcher Mindy Kurzer, University of Minnesota, "'are thousands of times weaker than natural estrogen. But they also circulate in the blood at levels thousands of times higher than natural estrogen.'"[97] The net result is that, even in micro-amounts (very small quantities such as found in real, natural foods), they offer a beneficial effect.

Some researchers are showing us that lower incidents in menopause-related symptoms in Asia may be directly related to diets containing greater amounts of phytoestrogen plants.

One report explains,

> After menopause, estrogen levels drop, and dietary sources of estrogen may have an important role in the female body. In Japan, where phytoestrogen rich soybeans are a common part of the diet (although only around 4-5 grams per day are eaten, on the average), only 10-15 percent of women experience menopause symptoms, where 80-85 percent of European and North American women (and who eat a standard western diet) *do* experience symptoms at menopause.
>
> In a recent study menopausal women were asked to supplement their diet with a phytoestrogen containing food—soy flour, flax seed oil, or red clover sprouts. The soy flour and flax oil (only) significantly prevented the vaginal mucosa from thinning and drying; but the effect of eliminating these foods caused the mucosa to return to the previous menopausal thinning and drying.
>
> In yet another study, post-menopausal women with bad blood fat profiles were split into two groups, with one group given bread and muffins made with flax seeds, the other group foods made with sunflower seeds. After six weeks, they switched seeds for another six weeks. The flaxseed lowered the 'bad' LDL

[97.] Schardt, David, "Phytoestrogens for Menopause," *Nutrition Action Health Letter*, January/February 2000, Volume 27, Number 1, Center for Science in the Public Interest, page 8–9.

cholesterol by 25 mg/dL (a 14.7% reduction) and levels of a protein called 'lipoprotein (a)', by 0.07 mm/L. Artificial estrogen
supplements lower levels of this particular protein, 'lipoprotein
(a)', but this is the first study to demonstrate that **diet can also
reduce the levels**, possibly due to [weak estrogens].[98]

Evelyn Leigh, Herb Research Foundation, explains, "Soy foods contain
phytoestrogens, compounds that have been shown to have both estrogenic
and antiestrogenic properties and that may help protect against certain
cancers, especially breast cancer."[99]

Soy foods, of course, are only one example of phytoestrogen-containing
foods. Nutrition writer David Schardt claims, "The food that is richest by
far in phytoestrogens is soybeans. A typical three-ounce serving of tofu,
for example, contains about 23 milligrams of isoflavones (the major group
of phytoestrogens). About a half-cup of shelled peanuts, on the other
hand, has less than a tenth of a milligram. Menopausal supplements made
from herbs like black cohosh, red clover, and dong quai may contain soy-
like levels of plant estrogens."[100]

It bears repeating that phytoestrogens simply are not to be found in
vitamin or multivitamin pills.

Although phytoestrogens are plant substances that mimic the female sex
hormones called estrogens, phytoestrogens won't turn any man into a
Marilyn Monroe look-alike. On the other hand, if you *are* a female, these
plant nutrients can help balance and regulate your hormonal system.
Phytoestrogens "may help relieve some of the symptoms of menopause and
lower the risk of osteoporosis, a bone thinning disease."[101] More than a

---

98. "*Hormone regulatory effect in women*", Natural food-Grains Beans and Seeds, The
Natural Food Hub, 2000 UHIS

99. ibid.

100. Lininger, Jr., DC, Schuyler, and Alan R. Gaby, MD, et. al., *The Natural
Pharmacy*, Healthnotes, Inc., 1999, page 426

101. ibid, p. 351

half million hysterectomies are performed every year in the United States as a means of resolving malfunctioning hormonal systems. Women should be made aware of their alternatives, because some medical doctors insist that 98 percent of these surgeries are unnecessary. Women should begin with their daily dietary intake to avoid hormone-disrupting substances because most diets today consist of foul nutrition that continues to harm and deplete the female hormonal system, creating imbalances leading to problems from irregular periods to hot flashes. Chief among the damaging dietary substances are synthetic and altered oils and fats, pesticide residues, chemicals/artificial ingredients, caffeine and refined sugars and flour. Phytoestrogen foods are helpful and should be incorporated into a real food-based diet that supports the hormone system rather than harms it.

Organosulfur

Organosulfur compounds are found in garlic, onions, leeks, shallots, chives and other so-called "sulfur foods." Organosulfurs are not contained in vitamin supplements because they are, of course, food components. Garlic, as a whole food, is an excellent source of organosulfurs. Much study has brought to light the benefits of garlic and its unique properties, including its abilities to destroy bacteria and protect people from high blood pressure. Garlic is, of course, an ancient food and still widely used today by natural health care practitioners in cases of high cholesterol, atherosclerosis (artery disease), high blood pressure, athlete's foot, bronchiole infections (lung and respiratory diseases), recurrent ear infections, parasites and vaginitis. Its active ingredient is *allicin* and it contains other sulfur compounds as well.

"Three reviews of double-blind studies in humans have found that garlic can lower blood cholesterol levels in adults by approximately ten percent. Garlic has been shown to be as effective as the drug bezafibrate in lowering cholesterol levels…Several double-blind studies also suggest it can prevent atherosclerosis."[102] In addition, "Human population studies show that eating garlic regularly reduces the risk of esophageal, stomach and colon cancer...Animal and test tube studies also show that garlic and its sulfur compounds inhibit the growth of different types of cancer—especially breast and skin tumors."[103]

It is speculated that organosufur compounds play a role in cancer suppression by blocking carcinogens (cancer-causing substances) and not allowing cancer-causing changes to take place in cells.

Isothiocyanates

A salt of isothiocyanic acid, an isothiocyanate food substance, is found in the cabbage family and possesses sulfur compounds said to "protect against some forms of cancer. Sulforaphane is one example. Isothiocyanates seem to act on detoxification mechanisms, thus speeding up the inactivation and disposal of potentially harmful compounds like pollutants from the body."[104] In plain English, isothiocyanates help keep our bodies safe from toxins.

Essential Fats, Fatty Acids & Lipids

Despite what we hear on television ads and news reports, fats from real, whole foods are not bad, but actually absolutely necessary for human health and life. The biggest problems we humans have with fats is when we eat fats that have been altered from their original state via cooking, pasteurization, frying, hydrogenation, roasting and even spoilage (causing rancidity). Such alterations change the molecular structure of fats so they no longer are regarded by our bodies as friendly substances. An essential

---

102. ibid, page 426

103. ibid .

104. Ronzio, page 351.

fatty acid (sometimes called vitamin F) is a fat substance that we need to consume in the foods we eat.

Essential fatty acids are used by our bodies for transmission of nerve energy, production and regulation of hormones, liver and other organ health, muscle contraction, inflammation responses, health of the hair and skin, wound healing and much more. Plus, fatty acids are needed for certain vitamins to function, including the fat soluble vitamins A and E. Essential fatty acids are prevalent in nuts, seeds (flaxseed is an exceptionally good source), vegetables, raw dairy products and fish and fish oils.

There are some diseases and symptoms that specifically point to a need for essential fatty acids, including multiple sclerosis, psoriasis, dandruff, eczema and even PMS (premenstrual syndrome).

Although fats have been defamed in recent times by marketing messages aimed at the weight-loss and heart-healthy market, we must be careful to distinguish between "bad" fats and good fats (discussed in greater detail later in this book). Fats are absolutely essential for our cells to keep us alive. The role of fats in the body is vast and not to be taken for granted; and Nature provides fats in whole foods; not in vitamin supplements. Volumes have been published on the value and nutrient effects of essential fatty acids, but for the sake of this discussion on whole food complexes, we'll merely offer a glimpse into this most-celebrated food factor that is sometimes referred to as vitamin F.

Essential fatty acids, as implied by the name, are essential to human health, biochemistry, cellular health and physiology. They are involved in energy production, transmission of nerve impulses, cell membrane composition and formation, brain and thinking functions, transfer of oxygen from the air to the bloodstream, the manufacture of hemoglobin, skin health and hormonal function. We cannot survive in health without eating raw, natural and whole food fats.

Fats are found in both animal (such as butter, meat, fish and cheese) and plant foods (vegetable oils such as coconut, olive, flax, wheat germ, sunflower, sesame). However, in the modern diet, real, raw and healthy fats from foods have given way to altered fats—fats that have been changed in their molecular structure to unhealthy fats and oils via food processing, hydrogenation, cooking, barbecuing, synthesization and rancidity via oxidation (exposure to air, oxygen). Cooked foods are the mainstay of the modern diet, making adequate amounts of fats, in their original healthy form, a rarity. Even wholesome fats in raw milk and butter have all but disappeared from the diet as political influences (the corporate dairy industry, for example) have illegalized raw dairy products under the pretense that they are dangerous due to bacterial contamination. Raw dairy products contain *natural* fats, while pasteurized dairy products (because they are heated) contain *altered* fats. Claims that raw dairy products are dangerous because they may carry bacteria is a weak argument in light of the fact that raw dairy has been the staple and sustenance of human life for thousands of years. These foods are mentioned in the texts of various ancient religions as well as mythological accounts predating even our oldest religions.

Symptoms of essential fatty acid deficiency may include fatigue, dry skin, immune deficiency, chronic fatigue, chronic illness, hypochondria, liver disease, nervous system disorders, attention deficit, growth retardation, sterility and hormonal dysfunction, mental disease, gastrointestinal disorders and heart and circulatory abnormalities. Fat soluble vitamins (vitamins that break down into smaller components in fatty environments within the body) are dependent on fats for absorption and metabolism. In foods, essential fatty acids are found right along with their important vitamin cofactors (helper nutrients)—vitamin E is found in wheat germ oil, vitamin A is found in fish liver oil, vitamin D is found in dairy, etc.

Anthony's Textbook of Anatomy and Physiology states, "An essential fatty acid is one that the body cannot synthesize and that is essential for survival. One's diet, therefore, must include essential fatty acids."[105]

[105.] Thibodeau, Gary A., *Anthony's Textbook of Anatomy and Physiology* 13th Edition, Times Mirror/Mosby College Publishing, St. Louis, MO, p.42

Fiber

Fiber, also called roughage or bulk, is the part of a plant made up of cells forming plant walls. Fiber is found in fruit, seeds, nuts and vegetables. Research has shown that fiber is essential for health in human beings due to its ability to clean the gastrointestinal tract. This promotes health of the colon and increases our ability absorb nutrients, remove waste efficiently, remove excess cholesterol, and lighten the burden on all of our bodily systems. Newer scientific research now claims that inadequate dietary fiber contributes to heart disease, hernia, cancer, spastic colon, high blood pressure, gall stones, obesity and other diseases.

"In a study of over 40,000 U.S. middle-aged men, researchers have found that heart attacks were 41% less common among men who consumed at least 28g (grams) of fiber daily compared with men who ate less than 13g daily as typical of the usual U.S. diet. It is estimated that fiber-deprived men reduced their risk of heart attack by 20 to 44% for each 10g of additional fiber, without lowering their fat intake. The largest reduction was among men who ate wheat bran, which represents mainly insoluble fiber."[106]

You won't find fiber in a multivitamin.

Fiber can be explained as a thick, cellular structure that strengthens and supports plant structures, yet we as human beings cannot fully digest it. This means that fiber passes through our digestive tract while cleaning and scraping it in this most natural form of internal maintenance. The best image of fiber is that of the stringy thread-like portions of celery, or the hard-to-break-down skin of an apple.

Studies have shown that fiber is important for the health of our cardiovascular systems by clearing cholesterol out of the intestinal tract. Fiber foods are also cancer preventives due to their natural cleansing effects. Looking closely at fiber, we find that it contains *lignins* that help to protect

---

[106.] Ronzio, p. 175

and retain the structure of fibers. Lignin is not degraded by digestive enzymes or bacteria within the stomach, but rather passes all the way through the digestive tract intact. Lignin decreases the risk of constipation because it increases the movement of stools and binds to bile salts and cholesterol to move them out of the body. "Certain lignin constituents released by the intestine are modified in the body. Such 'animal lignins' apparently interact with tissues, weakly mimicking the effects of estrogen, the female sex hormone. Lignin may have a therapeutic role in lowering the risk of breast cancer."[107]

Folic Acid/Folate

Folic acid (folate) is also known as *folacin* as well as vitamin M. Folate is a B vitamin that plays an important role in processes such as synthesis of the DNA required for rapidly growing cells, including those of the gastrointestinal tract, blood and all fetal tissues.[108]

Folic acid is especially important in the formation of red and white blood cells and blood platelets. As a result of folate deficiency, anemia takes place. Therefore, pernicious anemia, macrocytic anemia (presence of giant red corpuscles) and sprue are greatly benefited by the addition of folic acid foods to the diet.

The complex system of converting, using, storing and releasing folate is dependent not only on the ingestion of folate, but also on many biochemical processes. A healthy intestinal tract is needed for absorption of folate. A faulty GI (gastrointestinal) tract may result in the loss of folate, leading to folate deficiency. One example of how the GI tract may become impaired is through alcohol abuse; thus making folate deficiency a common problem amongst alcoholics and many alcoholic beverage consumers.

Folate enzymes are active in cell multiplication. Because cells lining the GI tract are among the most rapidly renewed cells in the body, anything

---

[107.] Ronzio, p. 271

[108.] Hamilton, page 209.

that interferes with making new cells results in rapid deterioration of the intestinal/digestive system. This leads not only to folate loss, but also the inability to absorb other nutrients.

Sources of folate include leafy green vegetables, legumes, seeds, yeast, eggs, whole grains, wheat germ, brewer's yeast, mushrooms, nuts, lima beans, kidney, cauliflower and liver. Yet, again, if someone is eating folate-rich foods without a healthy digestive system, folate deficiency symptoms and disease may be present anyway. Such deficiencies have been seen in alcoholism, empty calorie diets, infants fed on goats' milk (low in folate), and in various diseases in which cell multiplication is forced to speed up— cancer, multiple pregnancies, skin-destroying diseases (chicken pox, measles), burns, blood loss, etc.

A deficiency in folate may result in the impairment of cell division and protein synthesis—"processes critical to growing tissues. In a folate deficiency, the replacement of red blood cells and GI tract cells falters. Not surprisingly then, two of the first symptoms of a deficiency of folate are a type of anemia and GI tract deterioration."[109]

Folic acid, in a nonfood, isolated supplement form, may potentially mask the effects of vitamin B_{12} deficiency, which is especially common among vegetarians. The risk of anemia and nerve damage has been suspected by the authors of a review in a 1998 edition of *Archives of Internal Medicine*: "While it is rare, there have been cases where folic acid has masked vitamin B_{12} deficiency and led to seizures in patients with epilepsy, zinc deficiency and incidence of cancer and malaria...The author of the study, Dr. Norman Campbell from the University of Calgary in Canada, suggests that if folic acid intake is increased, the lowest dose that would ensure benefit should be used."[110]

[109.] ibid.

[110.] *Vitamin News*, Sept. 1996; re: *Archives of Internal Medicine*, 1996: 156

Biotin

Biotin is part of the B vitamin complex family and is essential for energy production in cells as well as the breakdown of proteins, among other things. Scientists have noted that biotin plays a part in fighting artery disease, high cholesterol, ringing in the ears, low blood sugar, headaches and high blood pressure. Foods containing biotin include egg yolk, meats (beef), brewer's yeast, fruit, rice, soybeans, legumes and nuts.

Esters

Esters include plant fragrances, fruity flavors and waxes and oils. Greatly overlooked by many healthcare practitioners is the role of fragrances and flavors in our bodies' response mechanisms to real, whole foods. The smell of a lemon, for instance, evokes a physiological response by our bodies in anticipation of eating, beginning with salivation and stomach activity. Such a response is proof of our intimate, not fully explained, relationship as natural beings with the natural world of plants.

Esters play an important role in cellular formation and the use of certain food substances by our bodies' biochemistry. For instance, esters can bring simple sugars together with minerals to keep the sugar from leaking out of the cells.

Sugars

The word "sugar" brings mixed reviews, from horror to mouthwatering delight, depending on whether you're talking to a dentist or a baker. Some people think of sugar as a wonderful flavoring, while others see it is as a dangerous chemical. But there's more. While some sugars are man-made and cause diseases, deficiencies and all sorts of health-defying symptoms, some sugars are natural and healthy when consumed in their natural context in prudent amounts. Sugars occurring in whole, natural foods are carbohydrates that provide our cells with energy. Since these naturally occurring sugars are still a part of the whole food complex and are in relatively small quantities, they do not present the health hazard of isolated sugar products such as sucrose, maltose, corn syrup, high fructose corn syrup, dextrose, glucose, white sugar, refined sugar, fructose and other euphemisms for refined sugars that either have been extracted from the original food complex or have been created synthetically or substantially altered in a laboratory.

Many native peoples have consumed real, whole food sugars such as sugar cane and fruits since the beginning of history without significant impairment to health. On the other hand, refined sugars (including those mentioned above), lead to tooth decay, diabetes, hormonal irregularities, mineral deficiencies, chronic fatigue and hyperactivity. Some estimates tell us that the average American consumes about 140 pounds of refined sugar per year (and rising), which is more than some people's entire body weight! Even if people do not add sugar to their foods, it is wise to read food packaging labels, because sugar (listed under many different nicknames) is added to most refined food products such as ketchup, barbecue sauce, pasta sauce, breads, cakes, muffins, cereals, ice cream, drinks, juices, jams, jellies, snack foods, restaurant foods, etc.

Saponins

Saponins are found in plants and are cholesterol-like molecules that have the ability to mimic steroid hormones. Saponins are found in soybeans, chick peas, mung beans and kidney beans. Some scientific studies point to saponin as a valuable cholesterol-lowering food factor and cancer fighting agent.

Tastes, Aromas, Odors & Appearances.

Other traits of whole foods include their distinct tastes, aromas, odors and appearances, all of which play some role, whether fully understood or not, in their healing properties. We know, for instance, that when we merely

think about biting into a lemon we actually begin a process of wondrous proportions within our physiology, as our minds prepare our bodies for incorporating such foods into our systems. The same process does not hold true for vitamin or mineral pills because they are not foods. Therefore, they are not akin to our true nature as human organisms.

There is an appeal to the aromas, or smells, of whole foods that elicit physiological and biochemical responses. When we take a whiff of alfalfa, full of carotenoids and minerals, there is a much different physiological response than when we sniff into a bottle of beta carotene or potassium supplements. Our bodies know the difference between real foods and chemicals at the most basic level. As such, we cannot underestimate even the smallest features of real foods and their impact on our bodies, as foods are part of the same nature as we are.

Qualities & Properties

This is a very vague and intangible subheading in this chapter. The truth is that foods have an array of qualities and properties that affect our health in a positive way, yet we do not (yet) understand why or how; nor have all of these properties been defined or identified. For thousands of years, native healers have used herbs to heal all sorts of ailments. They learned to trust in the "secret" ingredients of nature. At this point in our modern science, we have identified many of these ingredients, including minerals, bioflavonoids, fatty acids, etc., BUT we have still not identified all of the components that lead to healing and vitality. Most importantly, scientists have not even come close to determining the vastness and breadth of the variables that comprise living foods. Nor have they yet determined all of the specific ingredients within nature's whole foods that affect our bodies in a healthy way.

Our modern scientific institution has been criticized by natural health care practitioners for ignoring the value of Nature's plants once scientists began extracting specific nutrients from plants and attempting to recreate

their properties in the laboratory, resulting in the creation and proliferation of drugs and synthetic vitamin pills.

Civilizations much older than ours have long recognized plant and animal foods for qualities and properties far different from our westernized,
scientific understanding. For instance, according to Chinese medicine, the
qualities and properties of foods take precedence over their ingredients. In
the Chinese systems of "food cures" and herbalism, foods and herbs are
used not because of their vitamin content, but because they are known to
be hot, cold, sweet, sour, spicy, pungent, warm, cool, etc. These properties
then are used to address health problems identified according to a system
of qualities such as dampness, dryness, hot, cold, etc. Dr. Henry Lu, professor and doctor of Traditional Chinese Medicine, Vancouver, Canada,
writes:

> There are two basic differences between Chinese and Western
> diets. First of all, Western diet focuses almost exclusively on diet
> for weight loss. Chinese diet is designed not only to help you lose
> weight but also to treat many other ailments, including hyper-
> tension, diabetes, common cold, gastritis, diarrhea, constipation,
> cough, hepatitis, psoriasis, common acne, eczema, and so
> on…When I have a headache, I want to know which foods I
> should eat to cure my headache and which I should avoid to pre-
> vent my headache from becoming worse…The second differ-
> ence between Chinese and Western diets: In Western diet, foods
> are considered for their protein, calorie, carbohydrate, vitamin
> and other nutrient content, but in Chinese diet, foods are con-
> sidered fro their flavors, energies, movements and common and
> organic actions. It works like this: If I feel cold in my body and
> limbs, naturally I like to eat something that will warm me; if I
> feel hot, something to cool me. If I have a weak stomach, natu-
> rally I like to eat something that will make my stomach stronger;
> if I feel my kidneys are weakening, something that will make my

kidneys stronger. Ginger will warm me, because it has a warm energy; mung beans will cool because they have a cool energy...To be sure, we can find nutritional information on foods in Western diet. For example, we know that red pepper contains vitamins A and C, but it does not tell us that it can warm us; we know mung beans contain some protein and carbohydrates, but not that mung beans can cool us; we know that black pepper contains some protein, but not that it can make our stomachs stronger...The essential aspects of Chinese diet in regard to foods are: the five flavors of foods, the five energies of foods, the movements of foods, and the common and organic actions of foods."[111]

The entire ancient Chinese system of health, predating our own westernized system by thousands of years, and used effectively right up to the present, is predicated on an entirely different way of regarding health and the healing properties of Nature's foods without the need to scientifically "discover" and identify these properties before trusting in their effectiveness and reliability. In comparison, the main problem with westernized medicine, then, may be summed up by saying that it reflects an inherent distrust of Nature and an ignorance of Nature's power to heal. Westernized, modern medicine puts more trust in the limited knowledge of scientists than in the limitless, dynamic and life-creating power of Nature. In this modern line of thought, unless the scientific community can prove specifically what a food or herb contains and how the particular ingredient works, then they dismiss it as having little or no validity in addressing our health concerns. In addition to causing and promoting disease, this way of thinking has also led to a rapid decline of the health of our environment for failure to recognize the intricacies, balance and wisdom of Nature and perpetual attempts

---

[111.] Lu, Henry C., *Chinese System of Food Cures,* Sterling Publishing, NY 1986, pages 13–14

to "improve," alter and interfere with natural phenomena (weather, seasonal planting, ecosystems, the course of rivers and streams, allowing the extinction of animal species, etc.).

Energy & Other Unseen Qualities

Henry Bieler, M.D., a naturalist medical doctor who authored the groundbreaking best seller *Food Is Your Best Medicine*, wrote:

> If there is no energy there is no life. The sole and ultimate source of this energy is the radiation of the sun. This, however, cannot be utilized as such to maintain life, for life would fail at night if this were the case. Therefore, radiant energy is packed into small parcels by the chloroplasts of the chlorophyll-containing plants. If the cell needs energy, it does not use radiation but unpacks those parcels of energy, called "foodstuff molecules."...It is apparent that energy is life itself and that for man, who is a mammal, the vegetable and animal kingdoms are the source—the only source—of life and energy. It must be remembered that the animal eats the vegetable, or eats the animal that ate the vegetable. But man cannot eat all of the plants and vegetables which carpet the earth. Some are beneficial and nourishing and energizing, while others are indigestible and some are even poisonous; a number are stimulating to the body, while others are relaxing. But man, whose body is composed of the mineral elements of the earth, must seek his nourishment—his life and energy—from these same elements transformed by water and sunlight into plants.[112]

When we engage in a discussion about food energy, we begin to cross the boundaries of science into the vast unknown. If we go too far, we enter

---

[112]. Bieler, MD, Henry, *Food Is Your Best Medicine*, Ballantine Books, NY 1965, pages 202–203

the realms of theory, speculation and illogic. But if we stick only to scientific proof, then we miss out on receiving the healing potential of Nature just because our scientists have not given a food their seal of approval.

Specifically speaking, some of the energy qualities of real, whole, natural foods can be proven empirically (through scientific method), while other qualities remain unprovable at this time. So how do we know they exist? We know by food's *effects*, or in other words, we know by the benefits foods have on us even when we cannot prove how the benefits come about. Some researchers believe that the energy of food has to do with the complexity of the food in which there are many components interacting and interwoven in a symphony of dynamic activities—enzymes, vitamins, minerals, microbes, light receptors, and so much more, all working together in harmony. Scientists know that chlorophyll and other plant parts actually attract and convert energy from the sun, then we consume this energy. Scientists have also taken "pictures" of foods (called chromatograms) and compared these to chromatograms of isolated vitamins, only to find completely different patterns of energy, proving, for example, that vitamin C ascorbic acid does not convey or exude the same energy pattern as a vitamin C-containing food such as a lemon. Living, vibrant, healthy plants and animals contain a life force which cannot be found in dead, cooked and isolated parts. The concept of "life force" is a fascinating premise the continues to fuel ongoing work in search of the healing and preventive capacity of foods.

When we think of any organism, which in this context is food, then we must consider the importance of its energy and vitality—the key factors in determining whether the food will be beneficial to our health. There is certainly a difference between just a vitamin (a chemical) by itself in a pill, versus a vitamin that is still held intact within its original whole food. The latter possesses the ability, imbued by Nature, to energize our bodies, nourish our cells in the most natural way possible, and promote our own vitality, healing and immunity. One of the most remarkable traits of life is its energy—seen and unseen—and, within this energy, the capacity to perpetuate life. Sometimes this energy is latent, as in the case of a seed.

Seeds hold within them the ability to generate new life; to sprout into new life forms. Indeed seeds that have been buried in ice during the coldest winters have thawed only to grow into a new, life-supporting plant. Squirrels and other animals instinctively understand this and carry on a synergistic relationship with Nature, burying seeds and nuts to allow these latent foods to manifest into whole foods by sprouting and germinating underground. At the most primal level, such animals are farmers, sowing seeds today in order to eat and participate in the perpetuation of life in the spring. The inherent, latent power that lies within Nature's mysterious foods is testimony to their energy and life-giving properties. These are the kinds of foods we must eat to stay healthy; these are the kinds of properties found in whole foods and whole food concentrates that are not found in vitamin, mineral or amino acid supplements.

My dog, who knows nothing about science, and cannot even read (as far as I know), still knows enough to run out onto the lawn and start eating the grass when he feels sick. He hasn't once asked me for an asprin instead. You may say, "Yes, but that's because he's a dog, and dogs aren't as sophisticated or smart as people, or else they would ask for drugs." My answer to this is: natural beings seek natural solutions to their problems because they are in harmony with Nature. Animal behavior is motivated in a large part by what psychologists term the "reptilian portion" of the brain—a portion that makes up a part of the human brain as well. Our failure to see life in such simple and natural terms, however, may at least in part be attributed to the fact that we also have a rationalizing part of our brain that overrides this reptilian brain, many times to our detriment. Although our rational mind has led to the greatest achievements, it has also led to deeds of evil, traumatization, wastefulness and complications beyond the ken of any other creature on earth. Our complex brains are double-edged swords, capable of both great destruction and great creativity. Looking on the positive side, we can say that we have the capacity to create our problems as well as to solve them, ideally through prevention and wisdom.

YOU DON'T HAVE TO
REMEMBER THE PARTS

There are seemingly countless nutrients and substances that are parts of Nature's whole, raw foods. Note that I use the phrase "Nature's foods" to distinguish between foods that are found in Nature versus foods that are manufactured. Foods in Nature include fruits like oranges, apples and pears; vegetables like carrots, zucchini, broccoli and onions; herbs such as echinacea, goldenseal and horse chestnut; and spices like nutmeg, cinnamon and cardamon. There are also foods that fit somewhere between herbs, spices and foods such as parsley, garlic and cinnamon. Such natural foods are grown in natural conditions, in soil, sunlight and water. Foods that are "manufactured" are not natural. These types of foods are found in most grocery food stores, supermarkets and even in health food stores. Manufactured foods are not found in Nature; they are altered from their natural composition in many possible ways, or they were never really natural in the first place, wholly created in a laboratory out of unnatural ingredients.

First, manufactured foods are cooked, processed, refined, altered and heated; they are also often infused with other substances and termed *enriched*, as vitamins, minerals and other substances are added during processing. Orange juice is not natural nor is milk if these foods have been pasteurized. Pasteurization involves heating with the intent of killing bacteria. In the process of pasteurization, important nutrients and other natural food substances are destroyed. Heating kills enzymes needed by our cells for chemical reactions and digestion; heating destroys vitamins and denatures (changes the composition of) fats and amino acids (building blocks of proteins). Most manufactured foods sold at your local food store are heated and may be referred to as dead foods.

Second, manufactured foods contain chemicals that are foreign to, and not found in, natural foods. There are many chemicals known to damage the cells in our bodies, some of which are carcinogens (cancer causing); others are unpredictable in their effects, still others become harmful as the mix with other chemicals in other foods and the environment. It is not illegal for such chemicals to exist in manufactured foods. Some chemicals found in manufactured foods are:

- Preservatives: chemicals that keep foods from spoiling quickly;
- Emulsifiers: chemicals that keep ingredients from separating (for instance, to keep the oil in peanut butter from separating from the peanut portion and floating to the top);
- Pesticide residues which exist in all kinds of foods, from cookies to potato chips. If the food is not organically grown, you are eating pesticides;
- Synthetic fertilizers used on crops to artificially stimulate crop growth;
- Dyes to make foods more attractive;
- Artificial sweeteners, which are chemicals made to taste sweet;
- Refined sugar, a chemical formed from processing sugar cane, grapes and other fruits;
- Separators, which are chemicals used to keep ingredients in foods from clumping together;
- Artificial flavors, which are chemicals made to resemble all sorts of flavors ranging from lemon to cherry;
- Thickeners to give foods more "body;"

- Fake fats and altered fats such as hydrogenated fats, partially hydro-genated fats, olestra, margarine and others;

- Genetically engineered foods created by huge corporations inter-ested in controlling the production and sale of all food plants on earth. Genetically engineered foods have been altered at the seed level and are untested for their effects on health and human disease. They have been allowed into production in the United States (although most of Europe has banned their sale and use) only due to the political and economic power of corporations standing to profit from monopolizing the farming industry.

Real foods come from real plants, not manufacturing plants. Manufactured foods make people ill because the cells in our bodies are not created to handle, process and utilize chemicals that are eaten in modern daily diets. Our bodies are made to utilize natural foods, not human-made foods that are dead, full of chemicals and create all sorts of health prob-lems. Manufactured foods do not contain any real vitamins because foods that have been manufactured or destroyed or altered cannot contain real vitamins; the real vitamins are killed in heating, exposure to air and expo-sure to chemicals used in processing.

Refined, Processed Food Takes Its Toll

Foods sold in plastic, boxes, cans, bags and packages meant to withstand sitting on a grocery shelf for months at a time are not natural; they have been processed or treated in some way so that they are not recognized by our cells as nutritious foods. At best we can use parts of such foods to live; and at worst these foods make us sick; they lead to diseases of many kinds.

Despite what television newscasters report, the main cause of illness in this world is due to poor, inadequate and bad nutrition, NOT diseases caused by bacteria, viruses, sneezing coworkers, dirty hands, mysterious germs or exposure to aliens. Without good, real, whole, natural food, you are keeping your body's cells from performing their functions of protection, immunity and vitality. To keep healthy, we need a certain amount of natural foods in our diets.

Is Politics Getting in the Way of Your Health?

To talk about nutrition and health care these days without exploring the dynamics of politics is like trying to eat an elegant dinner with our hands behind our backs. Like it or not, today's politics affect every aspect of the structure and efficacy of our health care system, as well as the reasons why people hold specific views about health, nutrition, eating, and supplements. Health care and nutrition are influenced by today's political agenda, dictated by the largest corporations involved in genetic engineering down to the individual's reasons for popping vitamin C pills and ignorance about Nature's role in nutrition. Political, educational and legal institutions (by skillfully influencing the public through the mass media) in this country directly affect people's ideas and beliefs concerning the causes and spread of disease, scientific research, the need for taking supplements, the lack of respect for Nature, reliance on drugs and surgery, and ideas about what is acceptable (and legal) in terms of health care practice.

Although it may be unpopular to say, even westernized religion plays a role in creating a negative view of all things natural, teaching us that we are less a part of Nature, and more a dominator of it, by divine right. Some religions overtly teach that to believe in the power of Nature is to practice evil because they equate naturalism with Nature worship. This equation stems only from fear and culminates in the destruction and abuse of Nature, which in turn, leads to our own downfall, as we depend on Nature—rain, water, trees, plants, animals, sun and energy—to sustain us. To truly embrace such a concept that Nature is evil is to deny our own constitutions, dispositions and heritage. We are a part of Nature, not apart from it. The ultimate state of our health hinges on realizing this truth and using it to sustain and nurture us. The continual bashing of all things natural, including the environment and real foods, is a clever, but evil, activity of polluting and destructive companies to keep the public from supporting environmentalism. Auto manufacturers, chemical producers and oil companies head the list in working diligently to defame the work and passion of environmentalists who are proving that people everywhere are suffering and dying of toxic-borne diseases. These anti-American corporations hide behind pro-American slogans and rhetoric, but their actions show that they are responsible for destroying our air, soil and water. We have to look to alternative media to discover their treachery, deceit and tactics.

Websites such as **prwatch.org, wri.org (World Resources Institute), sustainableharvest.com, greenpeace.org and projectcensored.org** are reliable sources for uncovering the facts about corporate deceit and destruction that affects us all. As consumers, we need to begin to make purchasing decisions at our grocery stores based upon whether the products we buy are made from companies that are causing our relatives to die of cancer. This is a serious consideration, because it is obvious that big corporations are interested not in our health, but in our money, despite their cute little cartoon commercials or advertisements depicting their polluting trucks tearing through our endangered forests. America is under attack, not by terrorists alone, but by corporations destroying our "spacious skies and amber waves of grain."

Policies & Decisions Motivated by Profit

As a result of politics, scientific studies and "findings" are often predicated not on the objectives of curing disease and eliminating suffering, but rather on profiteering. Here in America the pursuit of making money is an obsession—a national pastime yielding both good and bad outcomes. Many a noble outcome has resulted from inventors and scientists looking to make a better mousetrap. No doubt we have been uplifted by refrigerators, automobiles, surgical tools, construction materials, recreational equipment, emergency medical procedures and communications devices.

Such creations have benefited manufacturers as well as the general public. However, it is also true that many innovations are not all they pretend to be. Through high-powered marketing campaigns and mass exploitation, the general public is made to accept, believe, utilize and crave many things that are not really good for them, but which make certain manufacturers financially successful. In the health arena, examples include refined wheat, refined sugars, artificial ingredients, preservatives, genetic engineering, cloning, pesticides, and vitamins, multivitamins and most drugs. None of these things are natural; even if they are *from* nature, they are no longer contained within the whole, natural entity. When we are told that unnatural substances are life-enriching and life-sustaining, then the scales of balance are tipped away from the general public's right to good health and in favor of the manufacturers' right to a healthy profit.

In place of receiving the healthiest forms of a food, vitamin or any other product, we as consumers are more apt to receive from manufacturers items and substances which are easiest, most convenient, fastest, best preserved, most profitable and least expensive to produce and sell. The economics and politics of the day interfere with what is best for not only the seller, but also the buyer (patient, consumer). In this way, economics and politics frequently takes precedence over environmental and health issues. Clearly, there is BIG money in the vitamin business (as mentioned, vitamin and mineral supplement sales are $6.4 billion per year); and the goal of vitamin manufacturers is to sell lots of vitamins, not to educate the public on the difference between a synthetic vitamin and a natural vitamin still contained within the food complex. The overall idea seems to be to convince us that pills are superior to whole, natural, pure and raw foods—the nourishment that has sustained all life forms since the beginning of life on this planet. As long as people feel some sort of effect from a vitamin, and are convinced that they need this substance to the point where they will pay for a monthly supply, then manufacturers have achieved their goals. The health of the public is a secondary consideration, if it is a consideration at all. We too often forget that the cornerstone of modern economics, *caveat emptor* (buyer beware), should be applied to drugs, medical treatment, alternative health care and vitamins, as well as any other marketed product or service. We must become better informed buyers, scrutinizing labels and manufacturers' claims.

Studies performed on the successful use of vitamins, minerals and other individual chemicals are made on isolated (also called "fractionated") and synthetic substances rather than on whole foods. Why? Economics. The purpose of conducting scientific studies in our modern world of science-meets-big-business is primarily to determine and predict the marketability and profitability of a given substance. Independent and private institutions conduct the most publicized scientific studies pertaining to vitamins, minerals and other food components. For a study to prove that vitamin C ascorbic acid, for example, helps alleviate flu symptoms is to prove that we should purchase vitamin C pills, which we do to the tune of billions of dollars each year. Thus, to show that a vitamin "works" like a drug against symptoms equates to the ability to sell vitamins and make big profits.

In light of the prevailing economic picture, it is not difficult to imagine why studies on the nutrient properties contained within (and not fractionated away from) foods rarely make the headlines. Once we discover the wonders of a vitamin **still contained within** the food complex, who can make money on it other than food growers (farmers and grocery stores)? Synthetic and fractionated vitamins and minerals are much easier to manufacture, preserve and sell than real, whole, natural foods. Once foods and herbs are standardized (in terms of milligrams, micrograms, etc., by adding in isolated vitamins and minerals to the food or herb), scientists can predict their effect like any other drug-like, chemical substance, and promise results. On the other hand, with real, whole food, such predictability is implausible and dependent upon many factors ranging from symptoms to bioindividuality (see the chapter "Coming to Terms with Natural Health Care").

Breaking Away From the Drug Paradigm

In Nature, no two carrots, or oranges or potatoes will ever yield identical quantities of a specific vitamin or mineral. This fact of Nature is used to argue *against* the efficacy of whole foods in fighting disease, feeding cells and providing immunity. But the naturalist will understand that **the value of foods is not limited solely to vitamin and mineral content**, but rather the complexity and completeness of the food. To judge a food for its total content of vitamins is to work within the pharmacology paradigm, not the naturalist paradigm. Nature's foods are not created to yield megadoses of vitamins; this is a human-made, arbitrary concept that we must break away from to truly appreciate the value of whole foods and their intricate complexes.

Is It Pharmacology or Is It Nutrition?

In this modern era, the practice of "nutrition" is a rare occurrence. Instead of practicing nutrition—the study and application of foods and their effect on illness and ability to promote health, energy and vitality—, most "natural health care" practitioners, including nutritionists, medical doctors, dietitians and chiropractors, actually practice *pharmacology*, using not foods, but rather isolated chemicals (pharmacological agents) to address symptoms, diseases and biochemical imbalances. As a result, there is probably more to learn from a farmer using medieval tools nestled in the Hunza valley than you can learn from a modern-day practitioner of nutrition or medicine. Instead of studying foods and their properties as part of the whole "complex," the modern tendency is to study vitamins, minerals, amino acids and enzymes in the same way that a pharmacist studies and appraises various chemicals and compounds. In other words, vitamins, minerals and other substances are "aimed" at certain "targets" (symptoms) to create a certain effect. It does not matter to scientists in these studies whether the body is being nourished or drugged, because eliminating symptoms and treating disease is the ultimate goal, with little consideration for long-term side effects or a chain reaction of biochemical imbalances.

Practitioners of truly natural health care, on the other hand, argue that the most important question to consider for ourselves is not whether a vitamin or drug seems to work, but rather whether it works *naturally*, in accord with the principles of Nature, in harmony with the body's biochemical and physiological functions, without upsetting (unbalancing and causing a chemical chain reaction within) natural systems, in micronutrient amounts (as opposed to unnaturally high potencies or high doses) and as a substance conceived by Nature to rebuild a natural system (that of our own cellular structures).

SCRUTINIZING THE MEDIA: TRUTH OR CONSEQUENCES?

You may ask "What does a discussion of the media have to do with health care, vitamins, drugs and foods?" Glad you asked. The simple truth is that we as American citizens are no longer receiving information through our major media to help us make wise decisions about our health, disease, prevention and dangerous chemicals in our lives. We are being kept in the dark while we suffer. Just as the Church once controlled the media, religion and educational institutions, leading Europe into the Medieval period, today's giant corporations have now ushered in their own form of the Dark Ages through the ownership, creation and censorship of news. The only difference is, in modern times, people are entitled to secular education, giving us the false confidence that we actually are privy to the truth.

When exposed to the idea that natural health care and food can be agents of healing and prevention, many people wonder why they have never heard of such things on TV or in the newspaper. Often I have been asked, "How come you don't read about the dangers of drugs or the poisonous side effects of fluoride on television? Who is saying drugs and chemicals are bad—some left wing health nuts?" I have to answer, No, facts about environmental toxins and drug side effects are being reported by our leading scientists in medical and scientific journals, not by a handful of crackpots who lack credentials in fly-by-night newsletters! It's just that we have a little-recognized inherent conflict between the major media and their sponsors and the public's desire to be informed. Most scientists and doctors with life-saving, important health information are never heard through the major media. Their work and their voices are suppressed if they threaten the number one corporate mission: to make money despite the impact on human suffering.

What Went Wrong With Our Media?

For the longest time in this country, the public has gleaned its news from the mainstream media—television, radio, newspapers and news magazines. We have always considered these media as our partners in democracy—keeping us informed on issues that affect our lives, health and safety. We have trusted and relied upon our media to give us the unbiased truth. This is no longer the case now that the major media in America are owned and operated by a select few corporations. Professor Peter Phillips, director of a national team of journalists associated with Project Censored, explains:

> Since the passage of the Telecommunications Act of 1996, a gold rush of media mergers and takeovers has been occurring in the U.S. More than half of all radio stations have been sold in the past four years, and the merger upon merger that resulted in AOL-Time Warner-CNN has created the largest media organization in the world. **Less than ten major media corporations now dominate the U.S.** news and information systems. Giant companies, such as Clear Channel, own more than 800 radio stations. Ninety-eight percent of all cities have only one daily newspaper, and these are increasingly controlled by huge chains like Gannett and Knight Ridder. [bold lettered emphasis added]

How did we lose control over our national media that once represented the interests of the public? We remember fondly from grade school history lessons how the United States of America rallied the patriots behind the banner of free speech and freedom of the press. But the free press is not the same here in the 21st century. Author Noam Chomsky explains:

In earlier days, there was a vibrant labor-based and popular press that reached a mass audience of concerned and committed readers, on the scale of the commercial press. As in England, it was undermined by concentration of capital and advertiser funding; one should not succumb to myths about markets fostering competition. Unlike in most of the world, business interests are so powerful in the United States that they quickly took control of radio and television, and are now seeking to do the same with the new electronic media that were developed primarily in the state sector over many years—a terrain of struggle today with considerable long-term applications.

Now that megacorporations own and operate the national media, most news is nothing more than PR (public relations)—the biased voice of industry that is manufactured for publication and broadcast to promote corporate business:

> A study by Scott Cutlip found that 40 percent of the news content in a typical U.S. newspaper originated with public relations press releases, story memos, or suggestions. In 1980 the *Columbia Journalism Review* scrutinized a typical issue of the *Wall Street Journal* and found that more than half of its news stories "were based solely on press releases." Often the releases were reprinted "almost verbatim or in paraphrase," with little additional reporting, and many articles carried the slug "By a *Wall Street Journal* Staff Reporter." There is no reason to think that the situation has improved since or that it is much different at other papers. "Most of what you see on TV is, in effect, a canned PR product. Most of what you read in the paper and see on television is not news," says the senior vice president of a leading public relations firm.
>
> This tendency is especially pronounced in the electronic media. Some PR firms specialize in the production of prerecorded public

service announcements and "video news releases" (VNRs)—entire news stories, written, filmed and produced by PR firms and transmitted by satellite feed or the Internet to thousands of TV stations around the world...VNRs are used heavily by the pharmaceuticals and food industries in particular, which provide a steady stream of stories touting new medical breakthroughs and previously unknown health benefits that researchers attribute to oat bran, garlic bread, walnuts, orange juice, or whatever product the sponsoring client happens to be selling. A subtle touch is needed to make sure that the VNR looks exactly like real news. Sometimes VNRs will use narrators who have previously worked as on air reporters. That these scripted stories are actually cleverly disguised advertisements is well understood by the people who work at TV stations and networks, but is rarely mentioned within earshot or eyeshot of the news-watching public.[113]

As an informed public we not only need to be aware of *manufactured* news, but especially news that is omitted from the major media, including stories on toxic dumping, air pollution, the destruction of the environment, alternative ("clean") fuel technologies (hydrogen, solar, wind, hydro, etc.) that now exist, the dangers of nuclear power plants, deaths caused by legal drug use and the suffering caused by U.S.-manufactured weapons (especially if these weapons are killing and maiming our own sons and brothers). Such stories would, in the eyes of the media, be bad for business—shedding a negative light on—or producing competition for—media owners and sponsors that include pharmaceutical manufacturers, energy producers, auto manufacturers, chemical makers and weapons manufacturers. If you were General Motors and the noxious emissions from your cars were causing asthma and cancer in children in every major city, would you welcome a news story about the menace of

---

[113]. Rampton, page 24.

automobiles? Or if you owned the electric company spewing pollutants into the air and water, would you want television viewers to see a news report about how solar-generated power can make them independent of you and your price gouging? Instead of cleaning up their act and protecting the public, toxin-producing companies simply want to suppress the news and replace negative images with those of SUVs rambling through pristine streams or taking a load of children off to soccer practice—the same children who are suffering from the effects of deadly car and truck exhaust. Think about this before you buy your next vehicle. The electric car is now available; buy one today and show your children you care about their future.

Today the main goal of the media, like any other privately owned company, is to promote the interests of those companies who give the media financial support, including industries representing modern medicine, medical doctors, pharmaceutical firms, chemical manufacturers, fast food chains, nuclear energy, electric companies, and more. These are huge, powerful, influential, rich corporations with agendas that may or may not coincide with the public good.

Instead of reporting unbiased news and scientific findings, the media publishes only stories which are not in conflict with their supporters. This means that our top scientists, researchers and doctors are not being heard through the most public outlets—television and newspapers. Meanwhile, in our scientific journals, medical journals and special interest publications, articles of great public importance are being published, but never through the mass communications networks where most of us can discover them. When is the last time you've heard of a layperson reading the latest issue of *Journal of Biological Chemistry*? The public is not given the opportunity to understand important matters such as the dangers of fluoride and chlorine, nuclear waste disposal that causes cancer, chemical spills causing leukemia in children, the fact that more than 500,000 hysterectomies are performed unnecessarily each year, how many nations throughout our world are rejecting genetic engineering and cloning, and drugs that cause more side effects than health benefits. Such information appears in our most prestigious, specialized publications (*Journal of the American Medical Association, Journal of Orthomolecular Medicine, The Lancet, American Journal of American Health*, etc.) but not in the mainstream media. In a nutshell, our corporations and their paid researchers are being heard, but not our top **independent** scientists!

Journalist Peter Phillips, an activist against news censorship, writes, "By ignoring critical social issues, mainstream corporate media dismisses democratic values in the United States."[114] Phillips and other journalists representing major universities around the country have, for the past 25 years, published top news reports that the mainstream media have refused to publish, despite the tremendous impact such reports would have on our lives. The news articles that never make it into the major media address some of the most important issues we need to know about to live in health, prosperity and freedom. Yet, because they are in conflict with the agendas of big business, the public's right to know is plowed under by corporate America's will to censor and suppress the news.

Big Business: Our Interest or Theirs?

The general public's stand on health issues is mostly influenced by big businesses. The voice of corporate America is represented with little or no challenge in the mass media. Making big profits is the ultimate achievement, regardless of the means of obtaining these profits or how they are beneficial or injurious to the general population and the environment. This is why we cannot trust the major media for our welfare. The media is a source of corporate information and persuasion that no longer works as a healthy arm of democracy. "Today's PR industry is related to democracy in the same way that prostitution is related to sex. When practiced voluntarily for love, both can exemplify human communications at is best.

---

114. Phillips, Peter, *Project Censored*, Seven Stories Press, NY 2001, page 11

When they are bought and sold, however, they are transformed into something hidden and sordid." There is no longer a fine line between earnest attempts at corporate sales and the dissemination of corporate information. Now the line is wider than the hole in the ozone layer, as manufactured news, outright lying and deception, and suppression of the truth is the hallmark of today's "news" reporting.

Why do news stories tell us that illness comes from germs, bacteria, viruses and genetic tendencies? Mainly because this is good for business. There is one important fact that we must always remember; it is a difficult concept for most people living in America, but it is true nonetheless: The media (television, newspapers, major magazines) are big corporations that are in business for one main purpose: to satisfy their clients. The major media are PRIVATELY (not publicly) owned by big corporations that make profits by making their clients happy. Their clients are oil companies, nuclear power companies, automobile manufacturers, phone companies, internet companies, electric companies, food manufacturers, chemical producers, fast food restaurants, drug companies and military weapons manufacturers, to name a few. Therefore, **the goal of the media is to report positive news about their clients**, such as the benefits of drugs, the tastiness of manufactured foods, the wonders of modern medicine, the benefits of nuclear power and so on. Negative news stories, for instance, about the horrific down side of nuclear energy (radioactive waste, danger to the environment, etc.) would be bad for business. This is not to say that leading scientists, researchers and doctors are not reporting their findings to the media, but rather that the media are choosing not to report these findings to the public because the findings conflict with the media's agendas. For instance, if nobel scientists report that fluoride is dangerous and creates thyroid dysfunction, the media will not pass this information on to the public because corporations who are behind fluoridation of our waters and who are powerful enough to affect media coverage are more important to the media than is the general public. Similarly, the work of Dr. Peter Duesberg, one of the world's foremost AIDS researchers who claims that AIDS is not caused by HIV, is NOT published in the mainstream media—on television or in the newspapers—because his findings are at odds with the medical establishment and pharmaceutical industry. Duesberg was at one time one of the most respected scientists in the field of virology, but once he decided to challenge the drug and research communities, he lost his livelihood, his reputation and his future. The pharmaceutical industry contributes billions of dollars to the media in advertising and marketing, whereas Dr. Duesberg contributes nothing but his research—research that threatens the money-making scheme of anti-AIDS drug manufacturers. The Duesberg example shows that you are only a talented, intelligent and diligent researcher only as long as you support the goals of your employer. There is no reward for independent thinking when you are being paid to prove the benefits of drug usage.

Certainly we believe that it is our right to know about chemicals that affect our health as American citizens in the land of the free and the home of the brave, but our desire to know is overshadowed by the business outlook of the media that are owned by major corporations. We are not informed of the dangers of manufactured foods, that cancer is caused by chemicals in our food and environment, or that illness is related to bad diets and poor food choices rather than genetics and germs because such facts point fingers at the owners and sponsors of the media. This is politics.

Author and political scientist Noam Chomsky writes: "Media service to the corporate sector is reflexive: the media are major corporations. Like others, they sell a product to a market: the product is audiences and the market is other business (advertisers). It would be surprising indeed if the choice and shaping of media content did not reflect the interests and preferences of the buyers and sellers, and the business world generally."[115]

---

115. ibid, page 25

Peter Phillips explains that the media's "censorship" of news to benefit the public is not always even necessarily purposeful or a matter of conspiracy, but more a matter of prudent business practice based on the desire to protect and promote their financial supporters and advertisers. The media, like other businesses, continue to grow in reach and size, in an attempt to increase their financial bottom line and power. While this is considered "good business," we have to consider whether good business equates to the creation of a healthy society. There seems to be a conflict of interests, with the general public on the losing end of the equation. Phillips writes:

> Media consolidation is creating a new form of censorship in the United States and undermining democracy in the process...Censorship in the United States is seldom deliberate. Instead it comes stealthily under the heading Missed Opportunities. Mega-merged corporate media are predominantly interested in the entertainment value of news and the maintenance of high audience viewing/reading levels that lead to profitable advertising sales...a recent Pew Research Center poll showed that more than 77 percent of all journalists admitted that news stories that were perceived as important but dull are sometimes ignored. More than a third polled stated that news stories that would hurt the financial interests of their news organization often or sometimes go unreported.
>
> This structural arrangement is what censorship looks like in America today: not usually a deliberate killing of stories by official censors, but rather a subtle system of information suppression in the name of corporate profit and self interest. Corporate media censorship is an attack on democracy itself. It undermines the very fabric of our society by creating a highly entertained but poorly informed electorate.[116]

---

116. ibid, pages 37–38

When the United States was founded, the media represented the American people and the American spirit. Our newspapers were much more reliable sources of information for the common good. Setting an historical precedent, we built our fledgling nation upon the principles of Freedom of the Press, Freedom of Speech and Freedom of Information. These are very noble principles that made us different from other nations. Yet few of us realized that these freedoms are NOT synonymous with, nor do they necessarily ensure, truth in reporting, unbiased news coverage and full disclosure of events. While we seem to still have these freedoms, we have as a nation failed to recognize that now our news media—major television, newspapers and magazines—are privately owned by big corporations that are not bound to the principles of presenting unbiased, truthful reporting. To the contrary, their aim is only to report the type of "news" that does not interfere with the corporate objectives of their clientele and affiliates. So we cannot rely upon our media to give us the truth about chemical spills, radioactive waste in our rivers, medical waste on our shores, demonstrations against big corporate monopolies and control over world trade, or the dangers inherent in processed foods and genetic engineering. We are kept in the dark, although we feel we have the right to know and we are conditioned to turning to our media for help, support and information. But, like in a plot from the television show *XFiles*, little does the public know that the media are not only keeping us in ignorance, they are actually the perpetrators of our demise.

Now that vitamins are popular, we don't hear the truth about these either; we do not read about their negative side effects unless they interfere with drugs. But even this is diminishing, because now most of the vitamins sold in our country are manufactured by drug companies. This is the politics of modern life here in the free nations of the West.

EXPLORING TWO ISSUES
NOT DISCUSSED OBJECTIVELY IN THE MEDIA

There are thousands of issues and newsworthy reports that should have appeared in our national media, yet are censored—many of these affecting our health and lifestyle. Following are only two examples of issues affecting all of us, selected for review for the sole purpose of elucidating the fact that there are two sides to major issues that we as citizens have the right to explore. The first issue is regarding the use of fluoride in our water systems, sold to the general public as health-promoting, while actually causing disease and possibly death. The second issue is cholesterol and fats, as we explore the positive aspects of these substances that are never reported in the mainstream media.

News the Public Does Not Hear

THE GREAT FLUORIDE SCAM

The issue of fluoride in our water supply and its use at the dentist office has sparked decades of ongoing disagreement and outrage that has never been made public via our media. The use of fluoride as a health-promoting substance is unfounded, yet most Americans (as well as dental professionals) believe fluoride is a godsend. Not only does fluoride not promote health, but worse, it causes serious illness and death. Such is the finding of a wide number of scientific researchers and doctors whose voices have never been given a public forum to let the public know we are being scammed, scared, misinformed and poisoned by an industry that is so politically powerful that it has successfully forced the dental profession into backing down without a fight. Even worse, the dental profession actively promotes fluoride use, choosing to accept corporate "research" in lieu of actual scientific evidence.

The fluoride issue has been debated for decades now, with most dentists telling their patients that fluoride is important in preventing cavities.

On the other hand there are many leading scientists, including dental specialists who adamantly insist that there is no scientific basis for using fluoride, that it offers no protection against cavities, and there is definitely a health risk from mild to cancerous.

There is no doubt that fluoride dumped into water systems across America is actually toxic waste from the phosphate fertilizer and aluminum industries. Likewise, under the pretense of killing germs, nuclear waste is now being sold to the public as agents for irradiation of produce that ends up on our dinner plates. The practice of selling toxic waste to the public is a new low in industry public relations and marketing. And it seems to be working just fine as long "industry experts" can get away with telling the public that there is a magnificent health benefit.

Professor David Hill (Canada) provides some shocking research that not only questions the power of industry to get away with health-destroying practices, but refutes the blatant lie that fluoride is safe and healthy. He writes:

> Promoters of water fluoridation offer the lure of strong, healthy teeth and reduced dental bills as inducements for communities to fluoridate their water. Fluoride is also promoted for other tooth-related uses. However, even the promoters have scaled down the benefits claimed for water fluoridation and admitted the danger of fluorosis from toothpaste. For every study by promoters over recent years repeating old messages that claim undisputed water fluoridation benefits—particularly reduction of cavities, there are equally reputable studies showing little or no effect on cavity rates. Studies in mainstream peer-reviewed medical journals and government reports now document the fact that serious harms are associated with exposure to small amounts of fluoride-including hip fracture, cancer, and intellectual impairment. There is evidence that both individual and institutional fluoride promoters have stacked the deck, manipulated

experimental results, suppressed evidence that spoke against their view, and victimized or smeared those who spoke out against them.

When old ways and knowledge are increasingly found to be based on false premises, incompetence, bias and worse, it is important to reexamine the old claims, and to take account of the growing body of research that shows they are at best equivocal and at worst completely opposite to the truth, and based on vested interest.

Fluoride promotion often proceeds with no understanding of the scientific method and sometimes without even the ability to perform simple arithmetic. The most important US Congress-mandated study in recent times on the suspected connection between fluoride and cancer was subjected to a series of Public Health Service review stages that successively downgraded the results from the original independent laboratory study to the point where they were declared "equivocal" and largely ignored. The proven association of fluoride and water fluoridation with increased hip fractures and reduced bone quality has been denied or downplayed. Many other lines of investigation have been ignored or not followed up in an open-minded manner.

Medical ethics, morality, economics, legal and political issues have not deterred fluoride promoters in their efforts. Indeed, the problem has been declared a legislative matter, rather than under the jurisdiction of courts of law which might introduce such notions as ethics and reasonableness. The main beneficiaries from fluoride use are the big industries that find a profitable outlet for their otherwise embarrassing toxic byproducts. It is time for change.

…We should all like to have strong, healthy teeth, the "benefit" promoters of water fluoridation offer. Water fluoridation, they say, has been proven in literally tens of thousands of studies to be completely safe, to provide a reduction in tooth decay of anything up to 70%, and has never caused an adverse reaction at the "optimal concentration" of one part per million (1 ppm)—no allergies, no cancer risks, nothing. It is not just good for children's teeth, but for everyone's teeth-especially old people's, and it may even strengthen bones. Why would any sane person oppose water fluoridation?

The answer is complex, but can be characterized by five statements of fact documented, where appropriate, in the peer reviewed medical literature:

- If it works at all, the benefits are very much less than claimed
- It is strongly linked to threefold increases in hip and other non-vertebral fracture rates; there is growing evidence of other even more serious medical consequences
- A recent study showed evidence of intellectual impairment caused by fluoride
- There is clear evidence that promoters have stacked the deck, suppressed evidence, and victimized or smeared those who speak out against the practice
- Given a recommendation for medication, individuals in a free society have a right to choose whether or not to accept treatment, a right to expect properly controlled dosage and medical supervision, and a right to be told the truth. Water fluoridation abrogates these rights.

Much more information is available than is reasonable to present in this paper. However, the reader should gain some insight into the problems occurring in the debate on water fluoridation, and be able to decide for themselves whether the controversy is false or not. My own conclusion is that there are, at best, real unresolved and serious questions about the safety and benefit of water fluoridation and related uses of fluoride. The most recent evidence suggests it is not particularly beneficial, and certainly not safe. The most charitable interpretation that one can put on the situation is that old habits die hard, and the medical/dental establishment is slow to adapt to the realities of modern research, and fearful of losing both face and law suits if they admit they made a mistake.[117]

The International Society for Fluoride Research, as stated on their website, "was founded in 1966 with the purpose of advancement of research and dissemination of knowledge, pertaining to the biological and other effects of fluoride on animal, plant and human life. ISFR publishes quarterly reports in FLUORIDE, on the biological, chemical, ecological, industrial, toxicological and clinical aspects of inorganic and organic fluoride compounds." The reader is encouraged to see what scientists have proven regarding the damaging effects of fluoride by visiting the website fluoride-journal.com/01-34-1.htm. The Society offers numerous scientific studies showing that fluoride damages blood cells, the pancreas, brain function, liver and kidney health and much more.

Visit the website www.fluoridation.com and you'll read that "the health problems caused by fluoride in some other countries are well-documented and staggering. There are about twenty nations with health problems due to fluoride ingestion." The National Treasury Employees Union reports:

> The union first became interested in this issue rather by accident.
> Like most Americans, including many physicians and dentists,

---

117. Hill, David, "Fluoride: risks and benefits? Disinformation in the service of big industry. Professor Emeritus, The University of Calgary, Alberta, Canada, republished online. This paper was updated in August 1997 from an earlier version presented by invitation at the public forum on fluoride and fluoridation, sponsored by the Chemical Institute of Canada, and CADACT, held at the Petroleum Recovery Institute, 3512–33rd. Street NW, CALGARY, Tuesday September 29th 1992.

most of our members had thought that fluoride's only effects were beneficial—reductions in tooth decay, etc. We too believed assurances of safety and effectiveness of water fluoridation.

Then, as EPA was engaged in revising its drinking water standard for fluoride in 1985, an employee came to the union with a complaint: he said he was being forced to write into the regulation a statement to the effect that EPA thought it was all right for children to have "funky" teeth. It was OK, EPA said, because it considered that condition to be only a *cosmetic* effect, not an adverse *health* effect. The reason for this EPA position was that it was under political pressure to set its health-based standard for fluoride at 4 mg/liter. At that level, EPA knew that a significant number of children develop moderate to severe dental fluorosis, but since it had deemed the effect as only cosmetic, EPA didn't have to set its health-based standard at a lower level to prevent it.

We tried to settle this ethics issue quietly, within the family, but EPA was unable or unwilling to resist external political pressure, and we took the fight public with a union *amicus curiae* <u>brief</u> in a lawsuit filed against EPA by a public interest group. The union has published on this initial involvement period in detail.

Since then our opposition to drinking water fluoridation has grown, based on the scientific literature documenting the increasingly out-of-control exposures to fluoride, the lack of benefit to dental health from ingestion of fluoride and the hazards to human health from such ingestion. These hazards include acute toxic hazard, such as to people with impaired kidney function, as well as chronic toxic hazards of gene mutations, cancer, reproductive effects, neurotoxicity, bone pathology and dental fluorosis.

One of the most notable accounts on the bogus claims of fluoride benefits comes from New Zealand dentist Dr. John Colquhoun, a one-time advocate of fluoridation whose research forced him to reconsider his stand and then make a public statement about his findings on fluoride treatment. Colquohoun writes:

> I looked at the new dental statistics that had been collected while I was away for my own Health District, Auckland. These were for all children attending school dental clinics—virtually the entire child population of Auckland. To my surprise, they showed that fewer fillings had been required in the nonfluoridated part of my district than in the fluoridated part. When I obtained the same statistics from the districts to the north and south of mine—that is, from "Greater Auckland", which contains a quarter of New Zealand's population—the picture was the same: tooth decay had declined, but there was virtually **no difference in tooth decay rates between the fluoridated and non fluoridated places. In fact, teeth were slightly better in the nonfluoridated areas.** I wondered why I had not been sent the statistics for the rest of New Zealand. When I requested them, they were sent to me with a warning that they were not to be made public. Those for 1981 showed that in most Health Districts the percentage of 12-and 13-year-old children who were free of tooth decay—that is, had perfect teeth—was greater in the nonfluoridated part of the district. Eventually the information was published.

> Over the next few years these treatment statistics, collected for all children, showed that, when similar fluoridated and nonfluoridated areas were compared, child dental health continued to be slightly better in the nonfluoridated areas. My professional colleagues, still strongly defensive of fluoridation, now claimed that treatment statistics did not provide a valid measure of child

dental health, thus reversing their previous acceptance of such a measure when it had appeared to support fluoridation.

I did not carry out the instruction to tell people that teeth were better in the fluoridated areas. Instead, I wrote to my American colleagues and asked them for the results of the large-scale surveys they had carried out there. I did not receive an answer. Some years later, Dr John Yiamouyiannis obtained the results by then collected by resorting to the U.S. Freedom of Information Act, which compelled the authorities to release them. The surveys showed that there is little or no difference in tooth decay rates between fluoridated and nonfluoridated places throughout America. Another publication using the same data-base, apparently intended to counter that finding, reported that when a more precise measurement of decay was used, a small benefit from fluoridation was shown (20 percent fewer decayed tooth surfaces, which is really less than one cavity per child). Serious errors in that report, acknowledged but not corrected, have been pointed out, including a lack of statistical analysis and a failure to report the percentages of decay-free children in the fluoridated and nonfluoridated areas.

Other large-scale surveys from United States, from Missouri and Arizona, have since revealed the same picture: no real bene-fit to teeth from fluoride in drinking water. For example, Professor Steelink in Tucson, AZ, obtained information on the dental status of all schoolchildren—26,000 of them—as well as information on the fluoride content of Tucson water. He found: "When we plotted the incidence of tooth decay versus fluoride content in a child's neighborhood drinking water, a positive cor-relation was revealed. In other words, the more fluoride a child drank, the more cavities appeared in the teeth".

From other lands—Australia, Britain, Canada, Sri Lanka, Greece, Malta, Spain, Hungary, and India—a similar situation has been revealed: either little or no relation between water fluoride and tooth decay, or a positive one (more fluoride, more decay). For example, over 30 years Professor Teotia and his team in India have examined the teeth of some 400,000 children. They found that tooth decay increases as fluoride intake increases. Tooth decay, they decided, results from a deficiency of calcium and an excess of fluoride.[118]

Conclusions on Fluoride

Despite testimony and research by experts from medical doctors to biochemists and from dental researchers to toxicologists, fluoride continues to be force-fed to Americans in nearly every city without any regard to **proven** dangers and the destruction of human lives. Most major cities use fluoride in their water supplies—a form of forced, mass medication. This is one of the most powerful cases to be made for the triumph of private industry over public rights to health and information. The question that begs to be asked is why we are not told of the dangers of fluoride on the nightly news. The answer is because our media does not represent our public interest, but rather the interests of their owners, partners, associates, advertisers and supporters in corporate America.

CHOLESTEROL CONFUSION: AN ENTERPRISING IDEA

By now we have heard it so many times that people swear it's the truth: cholesterol is bad; it kills people. But what the public has heard about cholesterol is misleading, untrue, half true, and panic-provoking. The facts

---

118. Colquohoun, John, "Why I Changed My Mind About Water Fluoridation," *Perspectives in Biology and Medicine*, 41, 1, Autumn 1997

about cholesterol have been obscured, misrepresented and unreported to the demise of public health and peace of mind. There is one fact that is undeniable, however, and that is: Cholesterol "treatment" is the center of huge profits and a flourishing industry. The sales of cholesterol-lowering drugs are staggering, as well as the sales of fat-free diet food products. People are afraid that high cholesterol will kill them, or at least, give them a heart attack, stroke and clogged arteries. Much of this fear of cholesterol is unfounded.

Author Uffe Ravnskov, M.D., Ph.D. (The Cholesterol Myths) explains:

1. Cholesterol is not a deadly poison, but a substance vital to the cells of all mammals. There are no such things as good or bad cholesterol, but mental stress, physical activity and change of body weight may influence the level of blood cholesterol. A high cholesterol is not dangerous by itself, but may reflect an unhealthy condition, or it may be totally innocent.

2. A high blood cholesterol is said to promote atherosclerosis (the scientific name for arteriosclerosis) and thus also coronary heart disease. But many studies have shown that people whose blood cholesterol is low become just as atherosclerotic as people whose cholesterol is high.

3. Your body produces three to four times more cholesterol than you eat. The production of cholesterol increases when you eat little cholesterol and decreases when you eat much. This explains why the "prudent" diet cannot lower cholesterol more than on average a few per cent.

4. There is no evidence that too much animal fat and cholesterol in the diet promotes atherosclerosis or heart attacks. For instance, more than twenty studies have shown that people who have had a heart

attack haven't eaten more fat of any kind than other people, and degree of atherosclerosis at autopsy is unrelated with the diet.

5. The only effective way to lower cholesterol is said to be with drugs, but neither heart mortality or total mortality have been improved with drugs the effect of which is cholesterol-lowering only. On the contrary, these drugs are dangerous to your health and may shorten your life.

6. The new cholesterol-lowering drugs, the statins, do prevent cardio-vascular disease, but this is due to other mechanisms than choles-terol-lowering. Unfortunately, they also stimulate cancer in rodents.

7. Many of these facts have been presented in scientific journals and books for decades but are rarely told to the public by the propo-nents of the diet-heart idea.

8. The reason why laymen, doctors and most scientists have been mis-led is because opposing and disagreeing results are systematically ignored or misquoted in the scientific press.

The overwhelming medical reporting on the mainstream media is, of course, that high cholesterol levels in the blood lead to heart disease and damaged and clogged arteries. Certainly, concern about heart disease (also called coronary heart disease—CHD) is statistically justified.

> Heart disease is the leading cause of death in the U.S., account-ing for nearly 740,000 deaths each year (287 deaths per 100,000 population), and cerebrovascular disease (stroke), the third lead-ing cause of death, accounts for about 150,000 deaths each year (58/100,000) In 1995, the American Heart Association esti-mated that approximately 1.5 million Americans would suffer a myocardial infarction [lack of blood supply to one or more por-tions of the heart], and one third would not survive the event. Although mortality from heart disease has declined steadily over the past three decades in the U.S., the total burden of coronary

disease is predicted to increase substantially over the next 30 years due to the increasing size of the elderly population. The cost of medical care and lost economic productivity due to heart disease in the U.S. was projected to exceed $60 billion in 1995.[119]

It may be argued, too, that not only is the predicted rise in heart disease due to an increasing elderly population, but also because of dietary and lifestyle choices that are detrimental to the cardiovascular system and health in general. These choices include the consumption of altered fats and oils, smoking, drug usage (drugs cause side effects), environmental toxins and nutrient deficiencies caused by dietary foods that actually rob the body of nutrients and injure the organs and tissues (fake fats, artificial ingredients, dyes, refined sugar and flour products, ice cream, caffeine and pesticides, to name a few).

What is Cholesterol?

"Though cholesterol has the reputation of an unwanted, even dangerous substance, all cells of the body require cholesterol because it is an essential constituent (ingredient) of all cell membranes."[120] Cholesterol is a waxy substance found in food and created in the liver. Although cholesterol is called a killer, any biochemist or physiologist will be quick to tell you that cholesterol is one of the most important substances in our bodies, and that all human life would cease to exist without it.

All steroid hormones are formed with the help of cholesterol. Thus, cholesterol forms sex hormones and adrenal hormones and is used by the skin to form vitamin D. The liver converts cholesterol to bile salts which are used to digest fats. Cholesterol, because it does not mix with blood or water, has to be carried through the body in low density lipoproteins

---

119. "Heart Disease, Artery Damage and PCBs," WebMed 2001.

120. Ronzio, page 94.

(LDL) which are fat-and-protein substances. HDL (high density lipoproteins) scavenges cholesterol from tissues and takes cholesterol to the liver for disposal. Elevated levels of LDL are seen by the medical community as an indicator of circulatory problems, with doctors fearing resultant clogged arteries. On the other hand, a growing number of doctors are suggesting that the real problem with cholesterol clogging arteries has to do with the poor, damaged condition of the blood vessels, not the fact that cholesterol is circulating in the blood stream. Indeed, one of cholesterol's functions is to patch damaged, cracked and disintegrating blood vessels. It is sent by the body to make a repair. Therefore, to get rid of cholesterol does NOTHING to repair or prevent blood vessel damage. It's analogous to killing the messenger for bringing bad news. The repair of blood vessels begins with changing the dietary intake of nonfoods that destroy tissues while at the same time consuming specific nutrients that rebuild arteries and heart tissues, including vitamin A, vitamin B, vitamin C and vitamin E foods as well as foods that contain important minerals such as selenium, iron, magnesium, calcium, potassium, etc.

Cholesterol-Containing Foods

Dietary cholesterol exists in eggs, meat, butter, milk and cheese. In addition, the body produces its own cholesterol in the liver. Plants do not make cholesterol, so we don't consume cholesterol in vegetarian diets. However, plants contain fats, oils, waxes and lipids—all types of fats, some of which are healthful and some of which are not. Further, even though plants are "natural," their fats and oils can indeed be altered enough to be unhealthful. For instance, a healthy nut can be rendered unhealthy through roasting.

The main question regarding the cholesterol controversy is: Does eating fatty, oily and cholesterol-containing foods lead to high cholesterol and heart/arterial disease? Diet food manufacturers like to say Yes! without a second thought. Some doctors claim that fatty foods in the diet leads to high cholesterol (elevated amounts of cholesterol circulating in the bloodstream looking for arteries to clog) and heart disease, while others claim it does not necessarily create problems. However, in our media which shouts at us more persistently and louder than our doctors, we only hear the warnings about the dangers of fat-filled diets and the evils of cholesterol as an excuse to be medicated or to purchase fat-free foods and go on a "heart healthy" diet. Funny, though, we do not hear about the dangers of consuming margarine. Is this because margarine manufacturers support the media with advertising dollars, or because the Margarine Association is a financial contributor to the American Dietetic Association? What do you think?

The exact cause(s) or predictability of high cholesterol is not fully understood by researchers. What we *do* know is that cholesterol can block our arteries and restrict the amount of blood flow which causes serious problems such as stroke, heart attack and circulatory problems. Since cholesterol is always running through our bloodstream, the main concern is why some people suffer from cholesterol buildup in their arteries while others are not injured by cholesterol. Considering this fact brings us closer to a possible answer. It is said by many doctors, including cardiologist Dean Ornish, M.D., author of *Reversing Heart Disease,* that the real underlying problem is weakened, destroyed and cracked blood vessels that the body tries to repair using cholesterol as a patch. Eventually, too much cholesterol builds up on the blood vessel wall which leads to occluded (blocked) arteries which leads to heart attacks, stroke and cardiovascular disease. In this case, it is not cholesterol that is the *cause* of coronary artery disease, but rather cracked and damaged blood vessels that deteriorate due to diets full of nonfoods and altered foods that, first, fail to nutrify cells, and second, leach nutrients out of the cells. Thus, cholesterol is the *effect* of disease not its cause.

Since blood vessel walls depend on real, complex nutrients (for example, vitamins A, C and E as well as bioflavonoids, oxygen and a host of minerals), a lack of such nutrients in the diet can easily cause destruction of cells, notably those forming the linings of blood vessels. This leads many physicians to claim that we should place more emphasis on straightening out the diet than on seeking to get rid of cholesterol, since diet and lifestyle are the underlying cause, while high levels of cholesterol in the bloodstream is only the symptom.

Speaking of Fats

Every detailed discussion on cholesterol leads to the topic of fats and oils and their effects on human health. This is especially because doctors have linked the consumption of fats to levels of cholesterol. One affects the other, they say. But not always. The truth is that many native peoples, including the Eskimos, have been consuming large quantities of fats in their traditional diets for many years without signs of heart disease. And Native Americans living on the plains subsisted mainly on buffalo meat without succumbing to strokes and heart attacks. Not until these people began to meld with "civilization" encroaching on their territories did cardiovascular disease begin to rear its ugly head. Changing from their original diet of whale fat to altered fats, the Eskimos began to see a rise in heart disease and cholesterol troubles. There are other native peoples (Tibetans, Mongolians, Australian Aborigines, etc.) as well who have traditionally consumed fats without causing heart disease, with diets centering largely around raw butter, raw milk, raw fat, raw cream and other animal foods. So it appears that, even though the low-fat/no-fat food industry fails to do so, we must really make a distinction between good fats and bad fats.

To borrow a phrase from food fat researcher Udo Erasmus, there are "fats that heal and fats that kill." Some of the killer fats appear in the form of oils, while others are in the form of altered fats and synthetic substances resembling fats and oils. Good oils, for instance, are unrefined, cold-pressed organic olive oil and flaxseed oil. In addition to providing essential fatty acids, cod liver oil (another good oil) also provides vitamin A. A source of good fat is from raw (unpasteurized) organic milk and cheese products. A bad oil is one that has been altered by scientists, including hydrogenated and partially hydrogenated oil. Other bad oils and fats include margarine and fake butters, artificial oils, most fried oils, rancid oils, oils from most roasted nuts and seeds and charbroiled fats on meats made over the barbecue. Fats in pasteurized milk, yogurt, cheese and other dairy products are bad as well. Bad fats are "bad" because they are unnatural substances that force that the body is forced to eliminate. They also put a strain on certain organs such as the heart, liver, pancreas, and gall-bladder, as well as the digestive system.

Good fats and oils from foods are needed for a variety of important roles in physiology and biochemistry, including cellular health and function, energy production, longevity, metabolism of other fats, nerve conduction, brain health, healthy functioning of the joints, health of the hair, skin and nails, hormonal health, and emotional and mental functions. Healthy ("good") fats are even needed for the health of our hearts and cardiovascular systems. For instance, fats are needed for nerve transmission; and the heart must have electric energy to pump.

What makes a fat good or bad? This depends on a number of important questions: "What kind of fat is it? How has it been treated—is it fresh, has it been exposed to light, oxygen, heat, hydrogenation, water, acid, base or metals like copper and iron? How old is it? How has it been used in food preparation? How much was eaten? What balance of different fats do we get...If we get the right kinds of fats in the right amounts and balances, and prepare them using the right methods, they build our health and keep us healthy. The wrong kinds of fats, the wrong amounts or balances, or even the right kinds of fats wrongly prepared cause degenerative diseases that we call *diseases of fatty degeneration.* Other nutrients can also cause fatty degeneration, and so can *lack of* certain essential nutrients. We can reverse diseases of fatty degeneration by making appropriate changes in fat choices, preparation, and consumption, and by supporting those important changes with attention to other nutrients in our food supply."[121]

---

121. Erasmus, Udo, *Fats That Heal, Fats That Kill,* Alive Books, Canada, 1993, page 5

To Eat Fats or Not to Eat Fats:
Conclusions About Cholesterol

Fighting cholesterol is such a big business (sales of drugs, diagnostics, heart and cardiovascular surgeries, diet foods, diet therapies and book publishing) that it overshadows the real health issue: Modern diets must change to a more natural and healthful course.

The issue of fats and cholesterol is complex. Sadly, what we hear and read in popular media is a simplified explanation of how dietary fat affects our health, leaving people in a perpetual state of confusion. "Fatty degeneration involves many substances other than fats, oils and cholesterol. It is, therefore, absolutely essential that we understand the broader context into which the story of the fats that heal and the fats that kill must fit."[122] If you do not have the time or patience (as few of us do) to study the cholesterol picture from all angles, the best means of action to avoid heart and vascular problems is to change your diet and lifestyle habits to the most natural course possible. There is a wisdom to Nature that is beyond the comprehension of modern man; it eludes scientific researchers the most, because these people are looking too closely at things and failing to appreciate the magnificent tapestry of life rather than the threads. Our bodies are designed as natural organisms to harmonize with Nature and her foods. The further we remove ourselves from this design, the more we fall prey to more and more health problems.

Instead of eating for convenience and taste, we need to be eating first and foremost for health, healing and prevention. Altered, processed and artificial foods cause heart disease, and this is where we should put our attention if our concern is cardiovascular disease or any other kind of symptom or illness. "Most fundamental to health is the fact that *the entire human body is made from foods, water, air and light...*This simple statement is the basis of a

---

[122.] ibid, page 5

revolution that is sweeping the globe—the foundation upon which the entire field of work that links nutrition to human health is built. From this basic truth follows everything that is part of how we must understand human health and the products and methods we use to care for it."[123]

Lowering Cholesterol

If you are concerned about your cholesterol levels, here are some easy steps that will help:

1. Eat mostly (70% of your daily diet) organically grown raw fruits, vegetables, nuts and seeds. The key word here is "raw."

2. Eat more fiber (included in the above diet). Cholesterol sticks to fiber and is carried out of the body through the digestive system. "Soluble fiber from beans, oats, psyllium seed, and fruit pectin has lowered cholesterol levels in most trials."[124]

3. Do not eat altered fats and oils such as margarine, hydrogenated and partially hydrogenated fats and oils, fried oils, roasted nuts, fried fish, grilled meats or chips and other processed snack foods.

4. Discontinue eating refined sugars and eggs. "When cholesterol from eggs is cooked or exposed to air, it oxidizes. Oxidized cholesterol is linked to increased risk of heart disease...Egg eaters are more likely to die from heart disease even when serum cholesterol levels are not elevated."[125]

[123.] ibid

[124.] Lininger, page 80

[125.] ibid, page 80, re: Hertog MGL, Feskens EJM, Hollman PCH, et al. Dietary antioxidant flavonoids and risk of coronary heart disease; teh Zutphen Elderly Study, *Lancet* 1993; 342: 1007–11 and Hertog MGL, Kromhout D, Aravanis C, et al., Flavonoid intake and long-term risk of coronary heart disease and cancer in the Seven Countries Study, *Arch Intern Med* 1995; 155: 381–386

5.Increase the amount of garlic you eat. Some studies show that garlic may lower cholesterol, while other studies cannot reach the same conclusion. Yet, since garlic is beneficial in many ways to the body, until it is irrefutably proven not to work, it is a good food to consume.

6. Stop drinking alcohol and monitor your drug intake. Although some studies show that moderate consumption of alcohol may increase HDL ("good") cholesterol, it also has the potential side effects of causing liver damage, high blood pressure, destruction of blood vessels and cancer. Similarly, a wide array of over the counter and prescription drugs destroy blood vessel and tissue linings, as well as the liver, brain, kidneys and hormonal system. Recreational drugs have no sensible value.

7. Seek out psychological therapy, stress reduction techniques, meditation, physical exercise and relaxation exercises to address the mental/emotional causation that may elevate blood cholesterol levels.

The above seven suggestions will not only benefit people with high cholesterol, but also any other acute and chronic health condition.

THE MIND-BODY CONNEC-
TION:WHEN NUTRITION
IS NOT ENOUGH

Any discussion of physical health is incomplete unless it also involves mental and emotional factors. Just like the foods we eat, and all other things natural, we as human beings are also complex. That is, we are made up of interrelated parts, from cells to bones to neurons, that all work together to keep us functioning. Yet this only describes our *physical* selves. We must also delve into our emotional and mental selves, because these aspects of us are inseparable from our bodily health and functions. Thus, there is far more to human health than food, exercise and other physically-oriented pursuits. We cannot ignore our emotional and mental aspects and the role they play in promoting and ensuring good health. To appreciate and nurture every aspect of our complexity (mind, emotions and body) is to invite wellness and healing. Let's start with some thought-provoking questions.

Does our mental state affect our physical health, and do our physical illnesses create mental and emotional problems? Does your mother-in-law give you a great big headache? Does your father-in-law's anger at the world make you bite your tongue? Do taxes make your mind want to jump out of your head and run off to a tropical island? When you are really nervous, do you have butterflies in your stomach begging to be set free? Did you ever have a feeling in your gut that there was something wrong? Have you ever fallen asleep because you were so bored? There is a definite link between our minds and bodies and the health of each. It has long been recognized that our mental and emotional problems impact our physical health. Certainly, our physical health can wear down our mental and emotional health. If you have ever suffered from a chronic sickness, you know what I'm talking about, because along with long-term suffering comes frustration, anger, depression, fear, anxiety, lethargy, hopelessness, loss of motivation and more.

The Interplay of Mind & Body

Our bodies' relationship with our mind and emotions is so spectacular that the body is able to take a mental or emotional state and interpret it into a physical manifestation. The exact way we do this still defies scientific knowledge; it can be demonstrated, but not always proven. Today's mental stress can be manifested into tomorrow's ulcer.

Skin rashes are also common for people under intense emotional stress; so are headaches and neck stiffness. Stomach aches, excess gas, chest pains, profuse sweating, clammy hands, clamminess and muscular contraction are all common reactions to emotional and mental overload. Fear, an emotional state, frequently translates into a physical state, characterized by a racing heartbeat and increased supply of adrenaline—nervousness. The body and the mind/emotions are in tune, harmoniously working hand-in-hand. While even the most scientifically-oriented medical doctor will testify to this mind-body connection, few doctors reach beyond these most common of symptoms in their treatment modalities, beyond prescribing drugs to subdue or stimulate the emotions, or referring hard-to-treat patients to a psychiatrist. Research shows that more than 130 million prescriptions were written in 1999 for depression and mental health related symptoms at a cost of more than $8 billion.[126] Indeed, if we have too many physical complaints, doctors frequently dismiss our claims and label

---

126. Duncan, Barry, Scott Miller, Jacqueline Sparks, *Networker*, "Exposing the Mythmakers," March/Apr 2000

us hypochondriacs. Is this a sensitive "diagnosis," or does this lead to more frustration, anger and depression? Our total health needs can never be met, other than accidentally, when our minds and bodies are not considered as part of the same, whole individual patient.

Chronic Fatigue: A Clinical Example

In my clinical experience, I worked with a a number of people suffering from what the medical community labels "chronic fatigue syndrome," consisting of symptoms that include restless minds, confusion, anxiety, digestive difficulties, panic attacks, irritability, depression, exhaustion, rapid heartbeat, mental fatigue, abstract fears, mood swings, hormonal irregularities and more. From a merely *physical viewpoint*, these stated symptoms are related to vitamin B complex deficiency; the absence of adequate amounts of vitamin B complex-containing foods in the daily diet. Vitamin B foods allow us to handle stress, protect our adrenal glands, support our hormonal systems, produce energy in our cells, feed the muscles, build red blood cells, work in digestion and keep our hearts beating in normal rhythm, to name but a few functions. From an *emotional viewpoint*, many psychologists claim that these symptoms are the result of trauma. So, are people suffering from chronic fatigue syndrome experiencing an emotionally caused problem or a physically caused problem? Or both? We may look at the chronic fatigue issue as trauma that causes stress that leads to a vitamin B complex deficiency. Or we may just as easily say that a vitamin B complex deficiency fails to support our emotional and mental faculties, culminating in trauma. From a wholistic perspective, however, we cannot afford to take such a staunch position and ignore the complexity of the mind-body interplay. It is my opinion that the mind/emotions and body should always be regarded as an inseparable entity for as long as we are alive—both need to be nourished and considered in the bigger picture of health and happiness.

The patients who came to my clinic with the chronic fatigue syndrome label had all but given up on medical treatment, especially after having been told that they have no concrete, provable physical illness because none could be determined by medical testing. Therefore, these unfortunate seekers of health were dismissed as having a problem that was "all in their heads" and received drug prescriptions for depression and other emotional problems. This is a shame, because drugs are not the cure for emotional and mental problems associated with physical ailments or for the innumerable mental/emotional causes underlying physical illnesses. Drugs do not address the cause of any illness, only the symptoms. Then they lead to unpredictable side effects often forming bigger and more complicated problems than the original illness. Drugs are designed to suppress or stimulate physiological functions—to push the body through a problem and eradicate symptoms so people can "get on with their lives." In the best case scenario, drugs may stabilize a critically ill or injured patient. However, the overuse of drugs due to their convenience, availability and power, always makes them potentially harmful resulting from dependency, side effects, addiction and symptom-masking. What good is a drug to address your chronic headaches if the *emotional* trauma CAUSING the headaches is ignored? Or, how do drugs uplift your state of health when you still eat a diet of foul nutrition and chemicals? Or, why should you change your destructive lifestyle habits when drugs mask their negative effects so you don't notice how much damage you are doing to yourself?

Chicken-and-Egg Conundrum

Illness can be a chicken-and-egg conundrum, as the determination of cause and effect is unclear and interdependent, based on the complex relationship between the mind and the body. A physical ailment always contains an emotional/mental component; while an emotional problem manifests in physical dis-ease or symptoms. And, as stated, a physical ailment, especially when chronic and long-term, often leads to emotional and mental suffering. With this understanding of our own complex nature, it is best to recognize that the mind and body work together and cannot be regarded as independent from one another if you really want to create healing and prevention.

The line between what is physical and what is emotional or mental is very often blurred, as reflected in our vernacular. We are apt to say when we can't cope mentally that our "nerves are shot." Or when we have too much on our minds, we "can't sit still." When we've been engaging in intense problem-solving, you may claim your "head hurts." If we are extremely frightened, our "knees buckle." When we hear good news, we "breathe a sigh of relief." The most simple and direct of all our expressions linking the mind and body is "He makes me sick!" This is the nature of the mind-body relationship—married and hand-in-hand down the aisle of life with no chance of divorce.

Nutrients for Emotional Support

There are many nutrients that directly affect our emotions and thoughts, supporting brain function, nerve impulses and thinking processes. Among these are vitamin B foods—seeds, nuts, whole grains, yeast, butter, cheese, eggs, etc. But we should at the same time keep our eyes open to the importance of nonphysical nurturing as well. Even if we are suffering primarily from an emotional problem, you can be sure that we also need to address the nutritional needs of our bodies to support our emotions. On the flip side, we can never be so close-minded as to ignore tending to our minds and emotions with mental nourishment—through psychological counseling, reading, meditation, critical thinking exercise, drawing, painting, singing, musical expression, laughter, love, discussion, writing, creativity, etc.

WE ARE TOO INDIVIDUALISTIC FOR SIMPLISTIC REMEDIES

What is the difference between you and me? This is a deep and multilayered issue. Culturally and socially we may share many commonalities and agree on many issues, from perspectives on freedom to security, and from recreation to patriotism. Physically, we may share other traits. This is what allows us to coexist in the same world to one degree or another. When we take a closer look, we are far less similar than our five senses lead us to believe. Scientists have proven that fingerprints, eye prints and DNA make each one of us a recognizably different person, whether we are of different races or whether we are one of twins. When we speak of ourselves in terms of cellular structures, then the differences become even more apparent and pronounced. If we look very closely, we are as different from one another as any snowflake is different from the next one to fall to earth and blend in with the rest of the snow that all looks the same on the surface. If we recognize ourselves and our interrelationships as *dynamic* (always changing), evolving beings, we see that we are not even the same person from one moment to the next, as our cells constantly reproduce and die to form a new "I," without our conscious awareness of this happening.

Cellularly and physiologically speaking, we are not the same individuals we were a year ago. This notion is the meal of philosophers and religionists who search to explain the real nature of a human being, leading many to believe that we are much more than brains and bodies, but rather spirits and souls. Science cannot identify, define or capture in any way that which we call emotions, willpower, thoughts, dreams, feelings, intuition, likes and dislikes, creative impulses, interests, love, fear or ideas. Such things cannot be studied as objects, but only considered in terms of their effects. When a brain is dissected by a scientist, there can be found nothing called an idea or a preference for the color blue, chocolate chips or Fellini movies. These are all nonphysical aspects of human beings beyond the grasp of science and physical observation, but we know they exist. Science cannot prove everything—maybe not even those things that are most important to us in our everyday lives, such as our deep love for our children, our sense of justice, our religious preferences or even our sense of humor.

These nonphysical characteristics of our personalities make us all different. We are individuals in every way, no doubt. Yet when it comes to health care, people think they can base their own treatment on what works for their friends, what they read in a newspaper, or what seems to be a simple solution to a complex problem. Similarly, as complex individuals, how could we ever believe that a simple drug or vitamin is the key to our health and happiness? Or even a combination of drugs or vitamins and minerals? As we have seen, nutrition is a very complex issue, incorporating a vast network of interwoven nutrients, energies and food substances into its healing properties. Even the way we feel about these food substances determines, to some degree, their effect on our bodies. Simple solutions to complex problems only work on a limited basis, if at all, and never address the complexity of any individual's problems, symptoms and concerns.

If we think of drugs and vitamins alone as serious health care solutions, we are not thinking hard enough about the true nature of ourselves and our needs; instead we are falling prey to the magic bullet, wonder-drug mentality that is the product of mass marketing, not logical, natural health care. You are *not* the same as everyone else, so mass marketing does not befit your individual needs, concerns and problems. Mass marketing is convenient and acceptable to marketing departments of corporations with products and services to sell us, but it is not satisfying to our senses of "self." To achieve optimal health and healing, we must seek an individualistic, wholistic and customized solutions, not some generalized, shotgun approach to healthcare where we throw vitamins and drugs at our problems in some desperate attempt to make something work.

It is no surprise, then that the shotgun approach to natural health care seems to be the standard among consumers, with the prevailing but misguided philosophy of "It's good for me, so it must be good for you too."

Given the complexities and variables associated with each human body, and considering the interrelationship between the mind and emotions, when a patient seeks care, the doctor is seeing only the "tip of the iceberg." Since doctors are busy people who do not have the time and resources needed to understand in detail each patient, he/she is rarely able to treat you as an individual to the degree that is necessary to meet your needs. Not only does each individual have symptoms and diseases to consider, but also genetics, daily diet, childhood illnesses, emotional trauma, race, anatomical peculiarities, tolerances, age, sex, climate, chemical sensitivities, history of drug usage, tobacco and alcohol use, degrees of sexual activity, sanitary habits, exercise or lack thereof, vocation, hobbies (exposure to glues, resins, dust, gasoline, etc.), religious beliefs, innate fears, stress factors, response to stimuli, particular thinking processes, prejudices and biases, location and environment of residence (urban, suburban, noise, pollution, stress, dampness, dryness, etc.), digestive status, sleep problems, sleep duration, current drug usage (prescription, recreational and illegal), temperament, metabolism, attitude, innate fears, intellect and tastes. That's a long list, but it is still far from being complete. At a micro level, each of our trillions of cells is different and ever-changing. At a macro level, our bodies occupy their own space and go through the day experiencing life like no other body on the planet.

The number of variables, combinations and interrelationships that make up each individual are staggering. Like everything else that is natural, we as human beings are complex. In addition, we are *dynamic*—ever changing and evolving from moment to moment and day to day. How, then, can a doctor effectively administer a drug when the patient is seen once every couple of months (which is considered frequent by today's standards) and the doctor doesn't take the time (or have the time) to form a greater understanding of that patient's individualism? Perhaps this is why native healers, such as traditional Chinese, Tibetan, Japanese, Korean and Native American doctors, often insisted on living with their patients for a couple of weeks or more prior to suggesting any form of treatment. Only then could the herbs and foods used in the healing modality be customized specifically for the individual.

Consideration of the "wholeness" and complexity of the patient is essential to reaching optimal health, yet this notion often seems to be against the grain of westernized medical thought. Psychiatrist Carl Jung perceived this failure to consider the complex nature of humans as the "missing link" separating Eastern and Western thought. Like many scholars, Jung noted that too much attention to detail and the scientific method obscures the "big picture." As we delve deeper into any subject matter, there is the ever-present danger of forgetting that the reason for studying the parts is to better understand and appreciate the whole. Further, Jung understood that the scientific method, while serving a great and noble cause, is a limited discipline. By its own human-directed and constructed design and limitations, science is unable to encompass, bridge or even appreciate the unlimited, dynamic vastness and complexity of Nature. In attempting to "prove" and define everything in the natural world via the scientific method, science is severely limited in its scope and power. It is arrogance and tunnel vision to declare that Nature's healing and nutritive powers only exist if they have been, or can be, proven by scientific method. Jung writes:

> Unlike the Greek-trained Western mind, the Chinese mind does not aim at grasping details for their own sake, but at a view which sees the detail as part of a whole.

This grasping of the whole is obviously the aim of science as well, but it is a goal that necessarily lies very far off because science, whenever possible, proceeds experimentally and in all cases statistically. Experiment, however, consists in asking a definite question which excludes as far as possible anything disturbing and irrelevant. It makes conditions, imposes them on Nature, and in this way forces her to give an answer to a question devised by man. She is prevented from answering out of the fullness of her possibilities since these possibilities are restricted as far as practicable. For this purpose there is created in the laboratory a situation which is artificially restricted to the question and which compels Nature to give an unequivocal answer. The workings of Nature in her unrestricted wholeness are completely excluded. If we want to know what these workings are, we need a method of inquiry which imposes the fewest possible conditions, or if possible no conditions at all and then leaves Nature to answer out of her fullness.[127]

What's Wrong With Your Doctor?

Of course it can be argued that, at least by consulting with a doctor, we have a better chance to individualize our treatment, because doctors are educated and experienced in diagnosis and recognizing diseases and symptoms. They also understand physiology and anatomy. This makes doctors valuable, but we should never rely on them solely to resolve our problems. The doctor-patient relationship works best when the patient is part of the decision-making, education and feedback process that makes every mode of treatment potentially more targeted to meeting individual needs. The more information you give your doctor, the more he/she should tailor your treatment. And as a patient, the more you know about yourself, your

---

[127.] Jung, Carl, *Synchronicity*, Bollingen Foundation, NY 1960

symptoms and nature's solutions to health care problems, the less you need to rely on your doctor to rescue you.

The doctor-patient relationship in modern society is too one-sided, culminating in the doctor dictating to the ignorant (or presumed ignorant) patient the best course of treatment with no challenges or debate invited or appreciated. This lopsided approach is at the core of ineffective, painful and dissatisfying medical care at the hands of all kinds of doctors—allopathic and so-called alternative alike. By proactively getting back to Nature and understanding the complexities of life and health, we are able to direct our own individual health and recovery, making it the kind of personal matter that it is meant to be. Doctors should be resources, not impersonal dictators, autocrats, untouchables and heavy-handed administrators of like-it-or-not commandments foisted upon their intimidated patients. Doctors need more patience (pardon the pun) for the humanity in healing and prevention. And patients need to understand that, after building a lifetime of disease, their doctors should not be expected to take responsibility for healing them. Although this may seem harsh, there is some wisdom to the statement I once saw posted in a print shop: "A lack of planning on your part does not constitute an emergency on our part." Prevention through diet, education, exercise and lifestyle is good planning. Expecting your doctor to perform miracles is too much to ask.

What's Wrong With Scientific Findings?

Scientific research findings on drug and vitamin effectiveness is misguided, incomplete and off-track because they fail to address the issue of individuality and take into account the aforementioned factors of the complexities of human beings. This fact alone is one great argument against using a "one size fits all" mentality for supplement and drug usage, despite promising studies. It is also the loophole in every scientific study which can be thrown out based on inherently invalid premises.

It is common for scientific studies to have potentially important methodological problems that limit their interpretation. One example of this is evidenced by a team of medical doctors involved in the study "The Antioxidant Vitamins and Cardiovascular Disease: A Critical Review of Epidemiologic and Clinical Trial Data." While the supplements in this particular study may at first seem to hold promise against cardiovascular disease, researchers were careful to note that people who take antioxidants may also tend to be *more health conscious than those who do not.* This leaves researchers wondering whether the use of supplements is only a common-denominator among already healthier, or healthy-thinking, individuals, and to what extent the supplements alone should take credit for the health of their users. In this example, researchers noted

> …lifestyle and dietary patterns probably differ significantly between persons who use and do not use antioxidant vitamins. For example, in four of the larger studies…persons using antioxidant vitamins were, on aggregate and in relative percentages, 24% less likely to be current smokers, 29% more likely to exercise regularly, and 10% less likely to have hypertension than persons who did not use the vitamins. Persons using antioxidant vitamins also consumed less alcohol. These findings suggest that persons using antioxidant vitamins may have other health and lifestyle behaviors that reduce their risk for cardiovascular disease. The absolute difference in these behaviors is not large enough to significantly alter the risk reductions seen for vitamin E or vitamin C intake; in addition, these differences have been considered in most of the cohort studies we examined, either by stratification or adjustment in statistical models. However, such adjustment may be unreliable if these other variables were measured poorly (such as a single unreliable blood pressure reading). Moreover, it is impossible to adjust for unmeasured health

behaviors that probably exist, given the more healthy profile of persons using antioxidant vitamins.[128]

Astute and experienced health care practitioners have been witness to many patients' exclamations of the wonders of their supplements in arresting all sorts of symptoms while pondering that perhaps a lifestyle change had more to do with profound health benefits than just the supplements. For example, a patient complaining of monthly migraine headaches may pick up a bottle of the herb feverfew and begin using it religiously. During the next office visit she tells her doctor that her headaches are gone, thanks to the feverfew. But she forgets to mention that she got a new job and her marital problems were all worked out or that she gave up foods with artificial ingredients due to a magazine article she read—all possible causes of the headaches in the first place. Perhaps her mother-in-law moved to Alaska and left the rest of the United States a stress-free environment. To get to the root of our health problems and their solutions, we must take an honest, unbiased look at as many pieces of the complex life puzzle that play a role in recovery—from our relationships to stress factors, and from our daily diet to the kinds of supplements we take, and so on.

The Case of the Mysterious Rash

How complex and individualistic are our health problems? Consider this interesting case. I knew a middle-aged scientist who suffered terribly all winter from eczema-type rashes all over his arms and legs and went from doctor to doctor looking for relief. He tried a variety of supplements—herbs, vitamins and essential fatty acids—and lotions with no relief. Then one day, when the weather turned warmer, the man noticed that his skin eruptions went away. To make a long story short, the man discovered that

---

128. *Annals of Internal Medicine*: Online report 1999. "The Antioxidant Vitamins and Cardiovascular Disease A Critical Review of Epidemiologic and Clinical Trial Data. Prabhat Jha, MD, et. al.

his skin rashes were caused from the woolen suit he was wearing during the cooler times of the year. After his rash disappeared, as an experiment, he wore his woolen pants again, and within a day the rash reappeared. He stopped wearing wool and the problem never returned. If the man had merely stopped wearing his woolen suit without ever making the cause-and-effect connection, then his recovery could have been attributed to lifestyle change, a miracle or one of the supplements he began taking. He may have even been told by his doctor, since there was no medical proof of his malady, that he was suffering from a psychiatric problem. Such is the complexity not only of health, but also of lifestyle.

Consider the Intangibles

Linked to this discussion on individuality is the vast field of mind-body health care; considering the complex interplay between the mind, emotions and body, as discussed in the previous chapter. Those aspects of our health—even if they manifest as physical problems—that are not physical cannot be ignored, and must be considered equally as important to our physical state of health as any other kind of problem. For years, the term "psychosomatic" illness has carried with it a negative connotation. For some reason, people have no problem admitting that they have a headache, backache or a cold, but there is a great stigma associated with admitting to any kind of problem stemming from an emotional or mental cause. To admit such a thing is, in most people's minds, an admission of some sort of weakness. As a nation, for example, we have no problem electing a president who had a cocaine addiction (George W. Bush) or one who had a chronic back problem (John F. Kennedy), but when it came to the thought of electing a vice president (Edwin Muskie) who once underwent emotional therapy, the nation viewed this as a weakness that could not be tolerated. The fact that societies take such an adamant stance against owning up to the realities of emotional problems creates all sorts of other problems. We cannot ignore the importance of mental health, and that it is a natural facet of life on earth that must be openly discussed and accepted. To treat every emotional problem as a weakness is a sickness in itself—it is a sick way of thinking that inhibits our growth not just as individuals, but also as a nation and a world community.

The completely intangible influences over physical health stemming from mental stress, emotions and thinking processes are as important to consider as the daily diet. Some doctors will even argue that emotions and mindset have a greater impact on health than any other factor. Headaches, ulcers, muscle tension, bowel irregularities, blurred vision, stroke, cardiac arrest and skin rashes have been known to manifest from emotional and mental problems. To date, the exact effects such emotions will have on health remain real but unpredictable and, to a great degree, unprovable. To complicate all of this, the body, mind and emotions change day to day, season to season, and year to year, and even with weather patterns. For this reason, traditional Chinese medicine has based its prescriptions and advice not on symptoms, isolated complaints or scientific studies of the efficacy of pharmacological agents, but rather on *symptom complexes*—a complex assessment of an array of symptoms that tend to create an overall picture of health. This takes a lot of work, research, experience and dedication to the patient—unheard of in today's fast-paced, magic bullet society. But this approach to health care is at least more fair to the patient than the thoughtless, one-size-fits-all administration of a drug or vitamin pill.

In consideration of bioindividuality (the uniqueness of each individual), to suggest that 10 grams of vitamin C per day is good for everyone, or that there's a cure for all cancers, or everyone needs colloidal minerals, or everyone benefits from fluoride in the water, or meat is bad for everyone, is a dangerous, speculative and unscientific generalization. And so it is unwise to embrace every vitamin and drug fad that becomes en vogue year after year.

Fads & Marketing Hype Doesn't Fit

With enough marketing hype, as a society, we witness a stream of outrageous promises claiming that every new fad product is a panacea for all of our ills. Next, everyone starts to give advice on how to cure one another's ills, sharing pills, eyeglasses, vitamins, lotions, creams, salves and inhalers. This phenomenon of health care advice-giving that flies unchecked in the face of caution and rationality has never been so evident than in the case of Ritalin, the drug most prescribed for hyperactivity in children.

Ritalin & Hyperactivity

Ritalin is misused as a simple solution to everybody's hyperactivity and attention deficiency without regard to considering individuality. Parents with young school children can attest to the fact that teachers and other school officials (who are not medical authorities or doctors or nurses) have begun recommending Ritalin for behavior problems as if this drug were no more potent than the chemicalized chocolate chip cookies they use as treats for good behavior. The resolution of hyperactivity, as with other health conditions, begs to be conveniently addressed with drugs rather than looking into the complexity of other factors that may be involved in the problem, whether mental, emotional, cultural, social, political or physical.

Is every child's attention deficit disorder due to the same cause? No, it isn't. Why, then, does the modern medical community treat it with the same drug? The astute doctor or researcher can name several, if not many, possible causes for so-called hyperactive behavior. Some of these include emotional trauma, excessive environmental stimulation (television, movies, computers, music, parental stress, etc.), poor diets (refined grains, refined sugars, preservatives, artificial ingredients), a fast-paced society that makes a classroom slow and boring by comparison, inadequate sleep and disrupted sleep patterns, and environmental toxins.

Some researchers, such as Albert Burgstahler, Ph.D. (Harvard University, Organic Chemistry), point to the damaging effects of fluoride on human biochemistry as a possible cause of ADD (attention deficit disorder). Burgstahler shows that one of the most notable effects of fluoride is impaired thyroid function, thus leading to hyperactivity in children and hypoactivity in adults.[129] Other factors contributing to hyperactivity may include deficiency in B complex vitamins, mineral deficiencies, learning disabilities, fears, mental distractions, boring teachers, the need for eyeglasses, and our electronic cyberworld that has outpaced the tedium of school work, to name a few. Rarely are all of the possible causative factors thoroughly exhausted before resorting to drug use because to do so demands an investment in time and observation.[130] Considering all of these things, the use of any drug without exhaustive investigation and research into each individual's complex case is a frightening approach to any health condition, let alone one that uses substances that have the capacity to cause side effects and nutritional imbalances.

The Misuse of Supplements

Like prescription and over-the-counter drugs, supplements of isolated vitamins, minerals, enzymes, and amino acids are also misused. Diet and lifestyle should be the doctor's first consideration prior to supplementation even with whole food concentrate supplements. Many health complaints disappear just by fasting (refraining from eating), radically changing to a raw food detox diet, increasing the amount of water we drink, getting rid of woolen clothing, following through with psychological counseling and therapy, moving out of a polluted environment, or learning to cope with stress. None of these solutions involves the ingestion of any supplement, drug or herbal extract.

---

129. *Acres, USA*, "The Fluoride Menace," March 2000.

130. An excellent review of Ritalin is discussed in *The Myth of the A.D.D. Child* by Thomas Armstrong, Ph.D., Penguin Books, 1995.

In a country where more is better, and the quicker the results, the better served, we have a dilemma that crosses the boundary from healthcare to conscience. Modern medicine is theoretically founded on the Hippocratic Oath whereby the doctor agrees to "first do no harm." This may be interpreted as a caution to be careful—to act with care for the patient. With the conflicting reports on the efficacy and safety and toxicity of fractionated and synthetic supplementation, certainly care must be the first priority. Because the body is so wondrously complex, there remains a doubt as to whether it can be simply treated with the use of isolates without creating biochemical imbalances and toxicity of unforeseen magnitude. Further, regarding synthetic vitamins, the naturalist may argue that no synthetic, unnatural substance has any place or use in the human body. Thus is formed the argument between chemistry vs. biochemistry.

Ruth Kava, Ph.D., Director of Nutrition, American Council on Science and Health, explains: Vitamins and minerals, frequently "used in pharmacological doses (doses much larger than could be obtained from foods)," are not monitored for their effects to any great degree because they are generally accepted to be safe. "Thus, these chemicals (**vitamins and minerals are chemicals**) may be sold without prior certification that they are either safe or effective for the purposes for which people buy them, and without scientifically established dosage levels for particular purposes."[131] "Those who do not support the widespread use of dietary supplements for either insurance or prevention are concerned about two aspects of the use of such products: safety and effectiveness…'Safe' does not mean completely safe for everyone under all possible circumstances, however."[132]

---

131. ibid.

132. Kava, Ph.D., R.D., Ruth, *Vitamins & Minerals, Does the Epidemiologic Evidence Justify General Supplementation?*, 2nd Ed., American Council on Science and Health, Inc., February 2000

We're Individuals, But We're Still Human Beings

Even in this highly technical, complicated, fast-paced world of the 21st Century, we are still just human beings. Although our technology, lifestyles and understanding of things in our world have evolved greatly, as human beings, physically and emotionally speaking, we have evolved very little over the past several thousands of years, causing our technology to overreach our innate abilities and temperaments. For instance, up until the last hundred years or so, a human being never traveled faster than thirty or so miles per hour. Now we race along at 80 miles per hour in our man-made metallic machines—automobiles, buses and trains—unnaturally and unsuited to our physiological and emotional sensibilities. Surely this must wreak havoc on our psyches as well as our bodies as we try to balance the natural limitations of our bodily systems with the speed, power, stress and potency of the world created by humankind's invention. Many doctors argue that, along these lines, even though we are little different physiologically from our ancient ancestors living in caves, our modern diet and lifestyle is wholly unnatural and destructive. In other words, we have not changed, but our diets have changed almost completely.

On the other end of the spectrum from the vitamin advocates, researchers studying the Paleolithic diets of our human ancestors are pointing out that the most primal biochemical and physiological needs of the body are to be found in natural, whole and unaltered foods. Some call such findings "science," while others label them common sense, because natural, whole, raw and unprocessed foods contain a complexity of nutrients that work harmoniously with the complexity of the human organism. Science's departure from Nature (and Nature's innate intelligence to create balance and feed all of the living organisms on earth) is in defiance not only of common sense, but also the essence of biology—a science in itself. Today's medical and scientific approach can only be related to Dr. Seuss' *Cat in the Hat* metaphor, wherein theoretical solutions lead to unseen problems which then create a problematic chain of events of unseen magnitude and predictability. Indeed, this is at the core of iatrogenic disease (illness caused by medical treatments) which begins with a health problem that is addressed with a drug that causes a side effect for which another drug is used, and so on, until now the cause of illness is the medical treatment itself.

The modern, Western-world diet in our so-called "advanced" countries is based on convenience, taste and economics, while, in contrast, the biochemistry of the body is based on nutrient requirements found only in natural foods. This makes modern man and woman in conflict with themselves, leading to the appalling disease rate that we have in modern societies. Despite all the drugs, vitamins, creature comforts, technological innovations and advanced food processing methodology (all unnatural), modern society remains plagued by diseases that continue out of control—cancer, tuberculosis, asthma, dental caries, diabetes, cardiovascular disease, arthritis and more. Ignored and swept under the rug are causative factors of disease that include environmental toxins, pesticide use, fluoride and chlorine additives, plastic degassing, nuclear waste, genetic engineering, mental and emotional stress, the overconsumption and/or misuse of drugs, and ubiquitous pollution of air, water and land. The return to Nature has never been more in demand for the salvation of humankind, the plant and animal kingdoms and the earth itself.

We have somehow lost our individuality in this fast-paced, chemicalized, quick-fix, electronic world of ours, so now our modern medical approach fails us. Instead of looking at patients as individuals with complex problems, doctors answer all health problems with drugs, surgeries and injections. It is no wonder why ancient forms of healing are coming back into widespread use—modern medicine is failing us as a society and as individuals with specific needs and problems. Gone are the days when the family doctor is a friend, confidant and healer from birth to death, generation after generation. This kind of doctor, now only remembered in Normal Rockwell paintings, has been replaced by cookbook approaches to disease. In other words, the patient comes into the doctor's office, explains his symptoms and walks out with a prescription or two, or three. If this doesn't work, surgery is indicated to remove "bothersome" tissues and organs. Indeed, it is not such a far stretch to say that the most widespread form of health care is not really "health" care at all, but rather *medical* care and/or drug management. The word "care" is really not appropriate at all. It only exists in advertisements, not in the hearts and practices of modern medicine.

Today's form of medical practice and marketing has been so ingrained in the national psyche that even so-called "natural" solutions to health problems utilize the modern medical model. The only difference is that people have begun acting as their own doctors. For example, we read that vitamin A is needed for the health of the skin, so we go out to the health food store and purchase a bottle of vitamin A palmitate and take as many as we guess may be appropriate. Sometimes the guess is based on a magazine article, sometimes on the recommendation of a friend. Shortly thereafter, our bodies undergo an internal chain reaction of biochemical imbalances that result in some other health problem that we never relate back to the first health problem that led to the ingestion of the vitamin A pills. And on it goes.

Health Investigators

All of this leads me to feel that real doctors should be called Health Investigators, because the way to better health is to explore as many variables as we can about symptoms and illnesses and their possible causes relating to the individual. The health investigator would also consider lifestyle habits, environmental exposure, diets and the other factors that influence health that were brought to light in this book.

Whole Food Concentrates vs. Vitamin Therapy

Regarding the issue of whole food concentrates versus isolated vitamin therapy, consider these words by food researcher Annemarie Colbin, founder of New York's renowned Natural Gourmet Cookery School for Food and Health:

> Nature—our nature—abhors an imbalance...Fragmentation affects foods not only on the cellular, but also on the chemical level. When wheat is refined into white flour, for example, not only does it lose its bran and germ, but some twenty nutrients are also lost or greatly reduced. Enriching the flour—which entails returning four of those twenty nutrients—does not solve the problem. Not only are the added nutrients fewer in number than those present in the original whole wheat; they also lack the **energy** they had when they were simply part of a living, growing plant. It's like cutting off your arm and then fitting you with a prosthetic one—it may have the same form and fulfill some of the same functions, but it is hardly as good as the original. Isolating the components of a living organism and then remixing them will not recreate the living organism.
>
> The logic, to me, seems obvious: *Added nutrients do not contribute to a live energy field.*
>
> In the ecosystem, the living creatures that comprise it are designed to subsist by consuming what the environment provides...Whole foods are simply fresh, natural, edible things, as close to their natural state as possible.[133]

Living in Harmony With Nature's Design

Unnatural, synthetic and short-cut solutions have been proven incomplete, inappropriate non-options for a diseased and decaying natural world. The key to recovering and promoting good health is to live in harmony with nature's design before it's too late. From the first days in

---

133. Colbin, Annemarie, *Food & Healing*, Ballentine Books, NY, 1996, pages 36–38.

school, our children should learn to appreciate their individuality, the innate intelligence of Nature, and the complexity of life. The other alternative is rapid destruction based on the delusion that we have somehow surpassed our own humanness just because our technology has reached elevated levels of advancement.

FOOD FOR THOUGHT: WHERE SCIENCE MEETS NATURE

By now we have seen that trusting in the innate intelligence of Nature and Nature's wondrous complexity is nothing short of embracing a philosophy that recognizes science cannot duplicate life or Nature, nor can it identify all of the nutritious properties of real, whole, raw foods. While scientists continue to create drugs and isolate vitamins, they cannot reproduce Nature's balance, dynamism, harmony and complexity. Just as scientists can create a robot to do the work of people, yet cannot reproduce human beings from a warehouse full of spare parts, scientists cannot create life itself. One of the hallmarks of life is its energy or life force—a poorly understood, elusive component that at its core cannot be identified. Nature's food is living food, a complex, energy-emanating substance that is harmonious with the human organism. When altered in any way at the hands of scientists, Nature's foods become unbalanced and infused with the potential to create imbalances and do harm. The introduction of chemicals, isolated vitamins, drugs and other inharmonious substances to the human organism creates unpredictable side effects and dis-ease.

As mentioned, we could call scientific and modern medical intervention "The Cat in the Hat Syndrome," referring to children's book author Dr. Seuss' infamous character whose interventions and attempted remedies only lead to bigger and more profuse problems. Using the Cat in the Hat model, for instance, the introduction of aspirin to relieve a headache may lead to a stomach ulcer that may be treated with a hydrochloric acid-quelling drug that may lead to chronic indigestion that may lead to unabsorbed vitamins and minerals that may lead to any one of a hundred symptoms resulting from malnourished organs and tissues. The more natural way to treat the headache would be to work diligently to uncover the cause rather than seeking to silence the symptom. The cause may be the overconsumption of fatty or mucous-producing foods, the use of drugs, the inhalation of toxic vapors, a neck, head or back injury, lack of blood flow to the head or even a congested or toxic liver. We must remember that headaches may be attributable to one of these causes, but they are never due to an aspirin deficiency! No human being suffers with a disease or a symptom due to a drug deficiency. So why does our modern medical industry persist in ignoring this obvious fact by insisting on drugging people each time they present a symptom? And why do we accept and embrace this irrational approach? What is the motivation for having our nation's medical system revolve around quick-fix, artificial approaches to health problems and disease—selling more drugs, selling more surgeries, selling more fad foods, selling more therapies, selling convenience, or all of the above?

Isolated chemicals, whether drugs or vitamins, always have a greater potential of causing further disruption of biochemical processes than Nature's well-balanced, nutritious foods. The main reason, as shown throughout this book, is because foods contain vitamins, but singular vitamins (even if several are mixed together in one pill) NEVER contain the rest of the food complex consisting of interwoven nutrients, energies and unidentified properties. This is not a philosophy, it is a scientific fact that is provable by examining the complexity of food substances as well as by studying the beneficial effects of foods in fighting and preventing disease.

The writings of Sir Robert McCarrison, M.D. ring as true today as when he wrote his milestone book *Studies in Deficiency Disease* in 1945, summing up all that has been noted in our treatise:

> [Vitamins] will be found to exist—and this is the important point—in the foods made in nature's laboratory, in quantities

and combinations adequate for the due digestion and assimila-
tion of the natural foodstuffs with which they are associated in
nature. The subdivision of vitamins into many classes is not
without the risks attendant on decentralization. Vitamins, like
other essential constituents of food, are not to be regarded as
independent of the assistance derivable from their associates in
the maintenance of nutritional harmony. Each vitamin is but a
member of a team, and the team itself but a part of the co-ordi-
nated whole.[134]

---

134. McCarrison, M.D., Sir Robert, *Studies in Deficiency Disease*, Oxford Medical
Publications, London, 1945, page 245.

APPENDIX A

OLDER STUDIES ON FOOD, VITAMINS & DISEASE

As we have seen, the concept of using foods to heal disease, build immunity and prevent illness is ancient and most likely prehistoric. In the least, even prehistoric man understood that he had to eat to survive! In the past sixty years, our modern society has seen a rapid and widespread conversion from natural health care and focus on whole food nutrients to an obsession with drugs and isolated chemicals (including vitamin supplements) to address symptoms and disease. On the simplest level, this shift was achieved because drug usage is easier to apply than persuading a busy, disassociated (from Nature) public to adhere to a sensible, health-promoting diet. On a more complex level, we know that drugs are big business, yielding huge profits that can be controlled by the medical establishment; foods, on the other hand, are easily accessible and allow for do-it-yourself health care. The obsession over drugs and isolated pharmacological agents, including vitamin products, (along with the resultant emergence of the multi-billion-dollar pharmaceutical industry's influence over medical procedures, health care choices, physician practices and the chemical approach to most disease and symptomatology) has obscured the impact of food studies and has overshadowed emerging medical findings about vitamins and foods in the 1930s and 1940s.

Thanks to the work of Dr. Richard P. Murray, clinician, biochemical researcher and food science writer, we can ponder some of these findings concerning the differences between isolated chemicals and food-based nutrients. In honor of Dr. Murray, who taught me much about nutrition and how to think about health care in terms of food nutrients and naturalism, I gratefully offer you his research so that his decades of hard work can be passed on to yet another generation. [135]

Different Vitamins Needed

"Attention is called by V.P. Sydenstricker, M.D., of the University of Georgia, School of Medicine, Augusta, to the fact that among human beings more than one vitamin is concerned in the production of any deficiency. The development of avitaminosis [deficiency of vitamins] is due to the failure or perversion of normal biochemical reactions which can be completed only when adequate supplies of different vitamins are available."[136]

Fish Oils & Diabetes

"The occurrence of increased amounts of carotene in the blood of patients with diabetes mellitus has long been recognized both by the clinical observation of xanthosis [yellow pigmentation] and by the results of laboratory tests. A group of 20 patients with juvenile diabetes mellitus were studied, and all were found to have poor light adaptation by the Frober-Faybor biophotometer. Three of the group were subjectively aware of night blindness, and nine showed cutaneous [pertaining to the skin] changes compatible with vitamin A deficiency. The daily administration of 60,000 USP units of vitamin A in the form of crystalline carotene dissolved in vegetable oil, for as long as 14 days did not affect the light adaptation of the patients with

---

135. Murray, Richard P., *Natural vs. Synthetic, Life vs. Death, Truth vs. The Lie,* Richard P. Murray, P.A.,1995

136. *Journal of the American Medical Association,* SocProc. 118, 12–1002, March 21, 1942

diabetes mellitus. The daily administration of 60,000 USP units of vitamin A to patients with diabetes in the form of **concentrated fish liver oils** caused their light adaptation to return to normal or nearly normal in periods ranging from 3 to 21 days. The cause of poor light adaptation in patients with juvenile diabetes mellitus appears to be an inability to convert carotene to vitamin A."[137]

Vitamin A in Butter

"…a unit of vitamin A in butter, determined chemically is apparently **more efficient biologically** than a unit of vitamin A in cod-liver oil determined in the same way."[138]

Vitamin B Factors in Yeast

"The addition of yeast or Peter's eluate to the diet regularly prevented this liver damage. Rich and Hamilton observed the development of cirrhosis of the liver similar to the Laennec type in all of fourteen rabbits which were kept on diet supplemented by various vitamins but lacking yeast. These investigators determined that the injury was due to lack of some factor contained in yeast other than vitamin B1, B2, B6 or nicotinic acid."[139]

White Flour vs. Whole Meal

"The nutritive value of straight-run white flour (73% extraction, tested on young growing rats) has been found inferior to that of whole meal flour, even when the defects of the former in protein, minerals and vitamin B1 have been corrected."[140]

---

137. Brazer, J and Curtis A, *Archives of Internal Medicine*, 1940, as abstracted by *Endocrinology*, 26, 5–936, May 1940.

138. Fraps, G and A. Kemmerer, *Texas Agr. Expt. Sta. Bull.* 560, 3–21 (1938) abstracted from *Chemical Abstracts*, 32, 8:3039, april 20, 1938

139. HA S., W., *Annual Review Physiology*, 3:259–282, 1941

140. Chick, H, *The Lancet*, 2:511–512, October 26, 1940

Stomatitis Study

"It (stomatitis [swelling and inflammation involving the mouth]) does not respond to treatment with vitamin B6, riboflavin or nicotinic acid, singly or in combination. Restoration of the mouth to normal was accomplished only after intensive therapy with the vitamin B complex. The factor or factors responsible are present in the vitamin B complex and may be any of the less well known fractions which have not as yet been isolated or synthesized and consequently have not been applied in human nutrition studies."[141]

Fortified Foods & Growth Rates

"I am very familiar with the difficulties involved with the fortification of foods with synthetic vitamins or concentrates are individual vitamins, and the results...clearly emphasize the problem in question. In this case chicks were placed on the modified Goldberger diet alone and supplemented with various synthetic vitamins and concentrates of some of the new members of the B complex. In most cases some improvement in growth was noted due to the feeding of each additional vitamin, but normal growth was not obtained until a fair amount of natural food such as liver, kidney or yeast was added. Likewise, **synthetic vitamins should be used with caution in order to prevent the development of deficiencies more serious than the deficiency we set out to control.**"[142]

Protein Diets vs. Supplementation

"In dogs fed a low protein diet supplemented with thiamin hydrochloride, nicotinic acid, riboflavin, pyridoxine hydrochloride and either pantothenic

---

[141.] Rosenblum, L and Jolliffe, N., *Journal of the American Medical Assn,* 117:2245, Dec 27, 1941

[142.] Elvehjem, C, *Journal of the American Dietetic Assoc,* 16, 7:654, Aug-Sept 1940

acid or purified liver extract, a deficiency state developed characterized by loss of appetite, substantial loss of weight, moderate to severe anemia and peptic and cutaneous ulcers. The condition was **prevented by an increase of protein diet**. [Disease was not cured or prevented by the addition of cystine, choline, paraminobenzoic acid, inositol or an eluate of clay absorbate of liver extract.]"[143]

Vitamin C

"I had a letter from an Austrian colleague who was suffering from a severe hemorrhaic diathesis. He wanted to try **ascorbic acid** in his condition. Possessing at that time no sufficient quantities of crystalline ascorbic acid, I sent him a preparation of paprika that contained much ascorbic acid and the man was cured by it. Later with my friend, St. Rusznyak, we tried to produce the same therapeutical effect in similar conditions with **pure ascorbic acid, but we obtained no response**. It was evident that the action of paprika was due to **some other substance present in this plant**."[144]

"It was demonstrated that guinea pigs fed vitamin C-free diets could be more thoroughly protected against infections with pneumococci by **lemon juice or orange juice than by pure ascorbic acid**."[145]

"The use of vitamin C when increased capillary permeability is due to deficiency of that vitamin is of course specific. **The fruit juices are more effective** than the synthetic vitamin C."[146]

---

143. Fouts, P., *Journal of the Americal Medical Assn,* Soc. Proc., 118, 12–1002, March 21, 1942

144. Albert Szent-Gyorgyi, *Oxidation*, pp. 73–74, Williams and Wilkins, Baltimore, 1939

145. Stepp, W, Kuhnau, J and Schroeder, J, *The Vitamins and Their Clinical Applications (Die Vitamine und ihre luinische Anwendung)* Ferdinand Enke, Stuttgart, Germany, 1936

146. Madison, F, comments by, on the paper of Fowler and Barer, *Journal of the American Medical Assn*

"Three cases of hemorrhagic intestinal disease did not improve after daily intravenous injections of ascorbic acid, but were cured by lemon juice…"[147]

"…treatment with natural vitamin C had reduced the incidence of typical paralysis by about on third as compared with the controls (from 92.8 to 59.1%) while the reduction of the two synthetic preparations combined was less than one-fifth (from 92.8 to 75.2%)."[148]

"In a speech before the Texas Pediatric Society in Dallas 1937, HC Poncer, MD, stated he had observed that 'frequently the hemorrhagic manifestations do not stop as promptly with pure ascorbic acid as with citrus fruit juices. The implication appears that possibly **the citrus fruits and natural sources of vitamin C** may contain something in addition to pure ascorbic acid which is important to the management of scurvy.'"[149]

"The group receiving ascorbic acid seemed to decline in weight much more rapidly and to develop more marked symptoms of avitaminosis than did action of an excess of vitamin C (ascorbic acid) on the metabolism as has been recently demonstrated by Mosonyt and Rigo. An excess of one vitamin may thus prove decidedly injurious."[150]

"One of the clinical tests for latent (early) scurvy is the measurement of the resistance of the capillaries (microscopic blood vessels) in the skin to rupture when the pressure within them is artificially increased by the application of external pressure. In human scurvy the capillary resistance is low. After crystalline vitamin C (ascorbic acid) became commercially

147. Lund, H and Elmby, A, abstr. from *Brititsh Journal of Chemistry and Phys.*, page 678, Aug 1938

148. Juneblut, C, *Journal Exp. Med,* 66, 4:459–4771, Oct 1, 1937

149. *Proceedings of the Texas Pediatric Society,* 1937

150. Grollman, A and Firor, W, *Journal of Nutrition,* 8:572–Nov 1934

available, it was found in many cases that the capillary resistance could not be increased even by administration of large doses of the crystalline vitamin. On the other hand, lemon juice appears to be effective in improving this condition. One group of workers interprets these findings as evidence that there is **another vitamin which is also important** in the prevention and cure of human scurvy. They do not dispute the necessity of vitamin C (ascorbic acid), but their contention is that this other factor, which they call vitamin P [now known as bioflavonoids] is **also essential.**

"Little is known at present regarding the properties of, or distribution of, this postulated vitamin P. It appears to be abundant in lemon juice and it is probably present in other citrus juices. Until the uncertainty regarding the actuality of vitamin P is removed, it is preferable whenever possible to use the natural antiscorbutic foods—the citrus and tomato juices and vegetables—rather than the pure crystalline vitamin."[151]

Vitamin D From Cod Liver Oil

"Ergosterol and yeast, when activated anti-rachitically by ultraviolet radiation, are inefficient sources of vitamin D for the chicken. Whereas 1% of cod liver oil of average potency resulted in normal bone production, it required from 40-120% cod liver oil equivalence as irradiated ergosterol and from 7.5% to 60% cod liver oil equivalence as yeast to produce the same results."[152]

"A chart taken from the work done by Mellanby indicates that in these studies vitamin D of viosterol [synthetic vitamin D] was probably less

---

[151.] Borsook, Nenry, PhD, MD, Professor of Biochemistry, California Institute of Technology, *Vitamins*, Viking Press, 1941, pages 109–110

[152.] Steenbock, H, S. Kletzien and J Halpin, *Journal Biol. Chem. 97:249, July 1932*

effective than the vitamin D of cod liver oil, in respect to the prevention of caries [cavities in teeth]."[153]

"A recent report states that the rat unit of natural vitamin D is about 100 times more potent in protecting chickens and children from rickets than the rat unit of irradiated ergosterol."[154]

"It is well known that the administration to children of irradiated ergosterol [synthetic vitamin D] meets with less clinical success than the older therapy of cod liver oil unless the unit dosage of the former is greatly increased over that of the latter."[155]

"The point was brought out that the relative effectiveness of the vitamin D of cod liver oil and the vitamin D of irradiated ergosterol varies with experimental conditions. Under the conditions of the present experiment, cod liver oil was fifty times as effective as the rat-equivalent amount of irradiated ergosterol for promoting calcification in the femurs of chickens."[156]

"Vitamin D factor in viosterol [same as ergocalciferol, synthetic vitamin D] and cod liver oil are not identical. Ten times as many vitamin D units in viosterol do not give as much protection as plain cod liver oil."[157]

---

[153] Mellanby, *Medical Research Council, Special Report Series*, No. 211, His Majesty's Stationary Office, London, 1936

[154] Supplee, G, S. Ansbacher, R. Bender and G. Flinigan, *Journal Biol. Chem.* 141, 1:957 107, May 1936

[155] Bunker, J and R. Harris, *New England Journal of Medicine*, 211, 25:1141, December 20, 1934

[156] Bills, C, O Massengale, F McDonald, And wirick, *American Journal of Biology & Chemistry*, 108, 2:323–330, Feb 1935

[157] DeSanctis, A and J Craig, *New York State Medical Journal*, 34, 16:712–714, 1934

"In rats, calciferol, the vitamin D of irradiated ergosterol, exerts greater toxic effects at lower levels than does the vitamin D of fish liver oil."[158]

Natural Concentrates are Complex in Nature

"'The Nutrition Committee of the National Health and Medical Research Council considered the proposal fully but decided that the addition of synthetic vitamin B1 alone to white flour involves a wrong principle. It is well known that there are many instances in which mixtures occurring in natural products have a **more beneficial effect than the administration of the isolated single substances**, e.g., in the treatment of pellagra, in which it has been found that, whereas the primary deficiency is of nicotinic acid, the best results are obtained by the administration of additional members of the vitamin B complex...' Instead it is recommended strongly that an investigation be made into the possible use as additions to the diet of products such as cereal byproducts [refined-out impurities] dried milk and other sources of the B complex rather than the use of imported synthetic products, since such byproducts would supply other known essentials besides vitamin B1."[159]

Wheat Germ & Yeast for Vitamin B Factors

"It was by no means certain that yeast extract or an extract of wheat germ which was very rich in vitamin B could be replaced, as far as the B complex was concerned by the synthetic vitamin. Some factors had evidently not yet been identified. Hence the reluctance to depend on other than the

---

158. Morgan, A, L. Kimmel, and N hawkins, *J. Biol Chem*, 120, 1:85–102, Aug 1937

159. *Journal of the American Med Assn*, Foreign Letters Section, 116, 9:882, March 1, 1941

natural foods. However, when a mixture of synthetic vitamins was combined, there was always **the fear that some essential factor as yet unidentified, might be left out.**"[160]

"In the present observations, these changes took place during a period when the intake of food containing vitamin B was inadequate and were relived by therapeutic agents (brewer's yeast and liver) known to be rich in vitamin B. Further identification of the substance liver extract responsible for the changes noticed must remain incomplete until various factors now grouped together as vitamin B are identified and separately tested."[161]

Treating Symptoms Without A Cure

"Nicotinic acid may aid in the restoration of health but among the pellagrins [those suffering from vitamin B3 deficiency] here described a considerable amount of ill health, such as anemia, underweight, diarrhea, and a few subjective symptoms, persisted."[162]

"It is obvious that pellagra, as it occurs in human cases, is a multiple deficiency. This seems only reasonable because of the close association of the various components of the B complex in their natural occurrence. It now seems clear from the work of many investigators that complete cure of pellagra will not take place through the administration of nicotinic acid [isolated vitamin B3] alone, particularly if the deficient diet is maintained."[163]

---

[160] *Journal of the Amer. Med. Assn.*, 118, 10:833, March 7, 1942, Professor J. Drummond, Scientific Advisor to the Ministray of Food, England

[161] Elsom, K and Sample, *American Journ Clin. Invest*, 16:4632, 1937

[162] Kooser, J and M Blandenhorn, *Journal of the Amer. Med. Assn.*, 112:2581–2584, June 24, 1939

[163] Gordon, E and E Sevringhaus, *Vitamin Therapy in General Practice*, The Year Book Publishers, Inc., Chicago, 1940

"Our investigations have shown that definite deficiency of vitamin B1 is not uncommon among hospital patients in England, and we wish to emphasize that **vitamin deficiencies in man are almost always multiple and are therefore usually inadequately treated by administration of a single pure substance.**"[164]

---

164. Goodhart, R and H Sinclair, *Biol. Chem.*, 132:11–21, January, 1940

APPENDIX B

QUICK & BASIC FACTS ABOUT NUTRITION & HEALTH

Vitamins, Foods, Nutrients & The Complex

- Nutrients come from natural foods we eat (as opposed to unnatural, processed and packaged foods) and are balanced within our foods to provide substances we need for health, vitality, healing and prevention. Vitamins are popular, but they represent only one category of nutrients out of thousands. This is why our bodies need much more than vitamins alone to be healthy. Foods and herbs are Nature's medicines, as well as clean air, water, sunlight and energy. We cannot survive on vitamin supplements, but we can survive on nature's foods.

- A vitamin naturally exists in a "complex," interwoven with other nutrients within food. The body knows the difference between a vitamin within its original food complex and vitamins which are synthetic or fractionated.

- Within a whole, natural food (or whole food complex concentrate), not only do you get the vitamins needed, but also all of the essential cofactors at the same time, including minerals, trace elements, amino

189

acids, proteins, enzymes, coenzymes, phytochemicals, lipids, antioxidants, bioflavonoids, carotenes, fiber, essential fatty acids and more.

- Chemists cannot make live food enzymes. Scientists cannot duplicate the complexity of natural foods; therefore, synthetic vitamins are not the same as food nutrients. Synthetic vitamins are not identical to vitamins found in whole, living foods.

- Separated from their natural components and synergists, vitamins may lose up to 99% of their use.

- Taking a combination of different fractionated vitamins DOES NOT equate to taking the same vitamins in a whole food concentrate supplement.

- People do not get all the vitamins they need from the typical modern diet.

- Ascorbic acid is NOT biochemically the same thing as vitamin C complex. Vitamin C, ascorbic acid, also known as a vitamin C supplement, is created synthetically from corn sugar. Real vitamin C, on the other hand, is found in whole, natural foods such as citrus fruits, berries and many green vegetables. Vitamin C is never found alone in nature; it is part of a whole complex of other nutrients ranging from minerals to enzymes and from bioflavonoids to pigments.

Enzymes

- One of the most important ingredients in foods and whole food concentrates is a vast group of substances called enzymes. Enzymes carry on many functions, from metabolism to digestion. There are many digestive enzymes that we need to help break down and utilize the foods that we eat, including ptyalin and amylase, which digest starches/carbohydrates; lipase and bile that split fats; and protein-splitting enzymes such as hydrochloric acid, protease, bromelain, papain, and others. Enzymes are types of proteins that act as catalysts because they enable and quicken biochemical processes.

The Impact of Refined Sugar

- When you eat refined sugar, many vital nutrients (including magnesium, potassium, calcium and phosphorus) may be pulled out of the cells and enter the bloodstream.

- Most sugar consumed in the American diet is refined/processed and may be a contributing factor in a whole array of illnesses including diabetes, tooth cavities, skin problems, attention deficit disorder, anxiety, hypoglycemia, hyperactivity, nervousness, lightheadedness, chronic dropping blood sugar, insomnia, overweight conditions, fatigue, poor appetite and indigestion, flatulence, skin diseases, respiratory membrane weakness, arthritis, tuberculosis, cancer, high blood pressure, fatigue, anemia, increased appetite, adrenal fatigue, PMS, chronic fatigue, chronic wounds/sores and more. For research on this topic, read *Lick The Sugar Habit*, by Nancy Appleton, Ph.D. (nancyappleton.com).

- Beware that refined sugars also go by the names of sucrose, corn syrup, fructose, maltose, powdered sugar, glaze, glucose, dextrose, lactose, sorbitol, xylitol, mannitol, caramel, dextrin, polydextrose, invert sugar, high fructose corn syrup, brown sugar, and even often "raw sugar." Any kind of sugar can be refined, not just cane sugar.

- Refined sugars can deplete the body of vitamin B complex; so can emotional/mental stress, drugs (prescription and illegal), birth control pills, caffeine, refined foods, chemicals in foods and environmental poisons.

- The liver is a "storage facility" for unwanted sugar in the body.

- Refined sugar is a drug, not a food. Sugar, like alcohol, is habit-forming. And refined sugar causes vitamin and mineral deficiencies.

The Politics of Media, Health & Disease

- All the news in the media regarding medical breakthrough drugs is NOT necessarily true. The major media of television and newsprint are no longer reliable sources of truthful, unbiased and trustworthy information because their goal is to appease their advertisers and corporate supporters, which include chemical manufacturers, refined foods manufacturers, pharmaceutical firms, fast food chains, the nuclear industry, etc. Top scientists and doctors are not being published in major media of television and newspapers because their findings are not in the best interest of the media's sponsors. This is the politics of big business as it comes face-to-face with the public's right to know.

Fatty Acids, Cholesterol & Bad Oils

- It has been estimated that approximately 80% of the American population consumes an insufficient quantity of essential fatty acids. Fat is a natural, necessary and essential component of food. Although portrayed as an evil substance, biochemistry shows that cholesterol, produced in the liver, is also essential for life and the function of cells.

- Cholesterol is a necessary part of every human cell and is imperative in almost every aspect of metabolism. High cholesterol is a symptom, not a disease. When synthetic or altered fats are fed to animals and people, they CAN cause cholesterol problems. Unnatural fats may destroy blood vessels.

- Cholesterol deficiency may lead to fatigue, obesity, nervous and emotional disturbances, digestive difficulties, impotency or inability to conceive and/or complete a pregnancy, menstrual syndromes and masculine traits in women, effeminate traits in men, blood pressure irregularities, fluid imbalances, nutritional deficits and imbalances and more.

- Blood cholesterol levels may be affected by genetics, underactive thyroid, mental stress and work-related tasks. Cholesterol can be increased by nicotine, pain, fear, pregnancy, lack of exercise, a number of drugs, and/or alcohol. Kidney disease, diabetes, hepatitis, and gallbladder obstructions raise cholesterol. And levels of cholesterol commonly increase with age. Cholesterol levels have even been known to change with the seasons.

- Good fats come from real, raw butter and milk (certified grade A), unprocessed (unrefined) oils such as extra virgin olive oil, raw nuts and nut butters, fish and good supplements of unrefined flax seed oil, borage oil, and wheat germ oil.

- Butter is healthier than margarine; margarine is not a natural food.

- Hydrogenated and partially hydrogenated oils are unhealthy substances which create an imbalance in the biochemistry. Hydrogenated oils such as those found in margarine, peanut butter and processed foods contribute to the destruction of the cells lining the walls of blood vessels.

Minerals

- Mineral supplements can cause a biochemical imbalance, leading to mineral deficiencies because minerals exist in delicate, intricate and synergistic relationships in the body. Therefore, for example taking iron, magnesium and calcium can inhibit manganese absorption. Too much magnesium can keep us from utilizing calcium. Excess iron, copper, nickel and other minerals can be toxic and impair other minerals in our bodies that we need, from zinc to phosphorus.

More than 600 Carotenoids

- Despite the popularity of beta-carotene as a supplement, there are more than 600 carotenoids in nature.

We All Have Our Individual Needs

- According to the principles of bioindividuality, it is NOT possible to design one daily diet that is perfect for everyone. This is also true of weight loss diets and supplement programs.

Vitamin B Deficiency

- It is best to consume whole foods containing vitamin B complex when suffering from exhaustion or fatigue. Such foods include yeast, whole grains, liver, seeds and nuts. Chronic fatigue with B complex deficiency may lead to adrenal fatigue.

- Symptoms frequently seen with B complex deficiency are unusual weakness and fatigue, insomnia, morbid fears, vague fears, indigestion from hypochlorhydria, apprehension, anxiety/a constant fear that something dreadful is about to happen, sweet craving, insomnia, confusion, rage and irritability. Beriberi (from vitamin B complex deficiency, especially thiamin) is the clinical disease, whereas all of the symptoms mentioned accompany the subclinical deficiency state.

Infectious Diseases or Deficiencies?

- In the case of so-called infectious disease, it is possible that the patient really succumbs to a nutritional deficiency, NOT to an infectious organism. Although most of us have been taught to believe that illness is caused by unseen germs, the fact is that most illness comes from nutritional deficiencies, poor diets, exposure to extreme/shocking temperature changes, and chemical poisoning in foods and the environment.

Food Refining, Pasteurization & Loss of Nutrients

- When whole wheat is milled into white flour, 83% of the nutrients are removed. The real purpose of processing and refining (food) is to increase shelf life, not to improve the quality of food.

- Natural forms of vitamin E [complex] lose up to 99% of their potency when separated from their natural synergists.[165]

- The health of the bones, cartilage, ligaments, tendons and joints relies on nutrients (especially minerals such as magnesium, calcium, phosphorus, manganese, etc.) from the diet. Sugar and acid-producing foods lead to arthritic pain, stiffness and degeneration. A main cause of osteoarthritis is from manganese deficiency. Mineral deficiencies are caused by a diet that depletes nutrients from our bodies, combined with diets that fail to provide nutrients in those foods we choose to eat.

- Pasteurization involves heating, which destroys (or greatly alters) nutrients (including enzymes) in foods such as milk, yogurt, cheese, cream and orange juice. Pasteurization denatures (changes the nature of) protein-like enzymes indigenous to milk. This means that milk that has been pasteurized no longer contains all of its enzymes. Because we need these enzymes to utilize milk's calcium, pasteurized milk (as opposed to raw milk) is not a great source of calcium.

Toxic Effects & Side Effects of Isolated & Synthetic Vitamins

Vitamin A

Acute intake of extremely high doses of vitamin A (>200,000 mg RE in adult humans) can cause nausea, vomiting, headache, and increased cerebrospinal pressure. Symptoms are generally transient. Chronic high

---

[165.] *Annual Review of Biochemistry*, 1943, page 381

intakes (e.g., >10x RDA) can cause hair loss, bone and muscle pain, headache, liver damage, and increased blood lipid concentrations. A particular danger in pregnant women is teratogenesis (birth defects). [166]

> As vitamin A is fat soluble and can be stored in the liver for long periods of time, it has a high potential for toxicity. The first sign of vitamin A overdose is usually headache, followed by chapped lips, dry skin, fatigue, emotional instability and bone and joint pain. There may also be hair loss, vertigo, vision problems, poor appetite, loss of weight, vomiting, liver damage and amenorrhea (cessation of menstrual periods). Individual tolerance to vitamin A varies widely and these effects can occur at doses over 7500 mcg RE (25 000 IU) although in most adults signs of toxicity occur with single doses over 75,000 mcg RE (250 000 IU) or smaller doses of 15 000 mcg RE (50 000 IU) taken for long periods. It is recommended that regular daily intake of vitamin A does not exceed 7500 mcg RE (25 000 IU) for adults and 3000 mcg RE (10 000 IU) in children. Pregnant women who take above 3000 mcg RE (10 000 IU) per day have a greater chance of giving birth to malformed babies. Vitamin A acne cream has been known to cause birth deformities and is now available only on prescription.[167]

[166.] Olson, J.A. (1994) Vitamin A, retinoids, and carotenoids. In: *Modern Nutrition in Health and Disease* (Shils, M.E., Olson, J.A. & Shike, M., eds), 8th ed., pp. 287–307, Lea & Febiger, Philadelphia, PA

Sporn, M.B., Roberts, A.B. & Goodman, D.S. (eds.) (1994) *The Retinoids*, 2nd ed. Raven Press, New York, NY.

[167.] Mills JL; Simpson JL; Cunningham GC; Conley MR; Rhoads GG. Vitamin A and birth defects. Am J Obstet Gynecol, 1997 Jul, 177:1, 31–6

Vitamin B1 Thiamine

In January of 1952, Royal Lee, DDS, wrote: 'I could write volumes on how synthetic vitamins like thiamine castrate the descendants of the victim who uses even as much as double the daily requirement.' In support of this statement, in a taped lecture, Dr. Lee cites a study by Dr. Barnett Sure (*Jol. Nutr.*, Aug, 1939). He tells us that Dr. Sure fed a group of rats twice the daily requirement of synthetic B. A like number of pigs were given the same amount of "natural" B. The results: All of the first generation offspring were sterile from the parents fed synthetic B. Obviously, synthetic B is not only not a nutrient, it is a genetic poison that damages the chromosome packages responsible for transmitting sexual characteristics from the parent to the offspring. In the case of Dr. Sure's pigs, the first generation offspring reaped the toxic, genetic damage. In the case of humans, more than one generation is required."[168]

"The symptoms of thiamin overdosing are similar to those of hyperthyroidism: 1. fast pulse; 2. irritability; 3. tremor; 4. weakness. Twenty to forty milligrams should not be used except in deficiency cases."[169]

Vitamin B3 Niacin

Toxicity: Large doses of nicotinic acid given to lower cholesterol may produce flushing of the skin, hyperuricemia, and hepatic abnormalities. These effects are reversed if the drug is reduced in amount or discontinued.[170]

---

168. Murray, D.C., Richard P., Natural vs. Synthetic, Life vs. Death, Truth vs. The Lie, p. 4, 1995.

169. Murray, D.C., Richard P., *Natural vs. Synthetic, Life vs. Death, Truth vs. The Lie*, p. 4, 1995 citing *Journal of the American Medical Association*, C. Mills, May 3, 1941; abstract in *Clinical Medicine*, 48, 9.231, Sept. 1941.

170. Swendseid, M.E., & Jacob, R.A. (1994) Niacin. In: Modern Nutrition in Health and Disease (Shils, M.E., Olson, J.A. & Shike, M., eds.), 8th ed., pp. 376–382. Lea & Febiger, Philadelphia, PA.

Vitamin B6 Pyridoxine

Excessive acute or chronic exposure to vitamin B-6 can be neurotoxic. It appears that in most individuals oral intakes of less than 500 mg/day can be tolerated. Larger intakes should be avoided. Because individuals may vary in their susceptibility to toxicity, a physician should monitor intakes in excess of the Recommended Daily Allowances (RDA) listed above.[171]

Vitamin C Ascorbic Acid

High doses of vitamin C may alter copper metabolism and lead to deficiency states. See Sources under Molybdenum.

In a study published in the April 9 issue of *Nature*, Dr. Ian Podman and colleagues from the University of Leicester in England found that vitamin C intake, at levels greater than 500 mg/day may not be advisable. These researchers studied 30 healthy individuals who were given doses of 500 mg/day for a period of 6 weeks. (The RDA for vitamin C is currently 60 mg/day). Results showed oxidative damage at the cellular level even after excess vitamin C was excreted. The authors of this study conclude that high doses of vitamin C may be doing damage to your cells as well.[172]

[171.] Leklem, J.E. (1990) Vitamin B6. In: Handbook of Vitamins (I.J. Machlin, ed.), 2nd ed. pp. 341–392. Marcel Dekker, New York, N.Y.

Raiten, D.J. ed. (1995) Vitamin B6 Metabolism in Pregnancy, Lactation, and Infancy. CRC Press, Boca Raton, FL.

[172.] Podman, Ian, Nature, April 9, 1998, (392:559) ; Eat fruits and vegetables. 5 a Day-for Better Health. National Cancer Institute. 1998

Hark, Ph.D., R.D., Lisa, Vitamin C: Its Role in Health and Prevention, 1998.

Vitamin D

Excessive quantities of vitamin D (in excess of 5,000-10,000 IU/day) can cause hypercalcemia, hypercalciuria, kidney stones, and soft tissue calcifications.[173]

Vitamin E

Very high doses of alpha-tocopherol-type vitamin E during pregnancy can cause birth defects.

Mineral Side Effects & Toxicity Molybdenum

High molybdenum intakes may increase copper excretion.

Iron

Excess iron can cause other metals such as copper, calcium and manganese to accumulate in the body by binding with them, and they become deposited in the wrong places and cause harm. Copper is notorious in this respect, especially if the liver is compromised. Manganese can also accumulate in the liver and brain. Calcium can build up in the arteries.

High intakes of iron increase the risk of heart disease. Too little copper, or too much calcium, may decrease iron availability. Further, according to author Elson Haas, M.D., Vitamin E "can bind the iron to a nonutilizable form, which then can oxidize and thus inactivate the vitamin E when the two are taken together, though this occurs more so with the ferric forms of iron. Ferrous sulfate has some interaction with E. The organic forms of iron—gluconate, aspartate, and fumarate—as well as chelated iron have little effect on reducing vitamin E. But, to be safe, it is best not to take vitamin E with iron but to take it by itself at night or in the morning."[174]

[173.] Holick, M.F. (1994) Vitamin D - new horizons for the 21st century. *Am. J. Clin. Nutr.* 60:619–630

DeLuca, H.F. (1988) The vitamin D story: a collaborative effort of basic science and clinical medicine. *FASEB J.* 2:224–236.

[174] Haas, M.D., Elson, Staying Healthy With Nutrition, 1997

A study published in the *American Journal of Epidemiology* suggests that men and women, particularly those over 60, are at increased risk of heart disease if they have high levels of iron in their diets. The study, which was conducted in Greece, involved 329 patients with heart disease and 570 people of similar age who were admitted to hospital with minor conditions believed to be unrelated to diet. Results showed that for every 50 mg increase in iron intake per month, men over 60 were 1.47 times more likely to have heart disease than their peers. In women over 60 the risk was even higher with a 3.61 fold risk for every 50 mg increase.[175]

Zinc and Copper

Zinc and copper compete with each other for absorption. Excess zinc intake for prolonged periods can lead to copper deficiency. Altered copper to zinc ratios may play a role in several disorders, such as heart disease, and some types of cancer, including those of the breast, lung and gastrointestinal tract.[176]

Acute zinc toxicity is characterized by gastric distress, dizziness and nausea. Symptoms of chronic toxicity include gastric problems, decreased

---

[175.] *American Journal of Epidemiology* 1998; 147: 161–166

[176.] 1 Schuschke DA. Dietary copper in the physiology of the microcirculation. Nutr, 1997 Dec, 127:12, 2274–81

2 Kremer JM; Bigaouette J Nutrient intake of patients with rheumatoid arthritis is deficient in pyridoxine, zinc, copper, and magnesium. J Rheumatol, 1996 Jun, 23:6, 990–4

3 Lukaski HC; Klevay LM; Milne DB Effects of dietary copper on human autonomic cardiovascular function. Eur J Appl Physiol, 1988, 58:1–2, 74–80

4 Knobeloch L; Schubert C; Hayes J; Clark J; Fitzgerald C; Fraundorff A Gastrointestinal upsets and new copper plumbing-is there a connection? WMJ, 1998 Jan, 97:1, 49–53

5 Jones AA; DiSilvestro RA; Coleman M; Wagner TL Copper supplementation of adult men: effects on blood copper enzyme activities and indicators of cardiovascular disease risk. Metabolism, 1997 Dec, 46:12, 1380–3

6 Serum copper/zinc superoxide dismutase levels in patients with rheumatoid arthritis. Mazzetti I; Grigolo B; Borzì RM; Meliconi R; Facchini A. Int J Clin Lab Res, 1996, 26:4, 245–9

serum ceruloplasmin activity and hypocupremia, decreased lymphocyte stimulation to PHA and reduced HDL cholesterol. An emetic (bringing or causing vomiting) effect occurs at >150 mg Zn/day.

Dietary supplements of zinc approximating the Recommended Dietary Allowance (15 mg for adults) and higher doses produce potentially harmful abnormalities of lipid metabolism by inducing mild copper deficiency.[177]

Selenium

Selenium toxicity is characterized by dermatologic (skin) lesions. Selenotic [selenium-poisoned] animals and humans develop brittle hair and nails/hooves. Sporadic cases of selenium-poisoning have been reported involving industrial or accidental exposures to selenium-compounds. In certain rural Chinese communities chronic intakes of very high amounts of selenium were linked to skin, hair and nail abnormalities which disappeared upon resuming regular selenium intakes. Selenium has been identified as the cause of birth deformities in migratory wildfowl in a wetland area (Kesteron Reservoir, CA) which receives selenium-enriched irrigation

[177.] Cousins, R.J. (1996) *Zinc. In: Present Knowledge in Nutrition* (Filer, L.J. & Ziegler, E.E., eds.), 7th Ed., pp. 293–306. International Life Sciences Institute Press, Washington, DC

King, J.C. & C.L. Keen (1994) Zinc. In: Modern Nutrition in Health and Disease, (M.E. Shils, J.A. Olson & M. Shike, eds.), 8th ed., pp. 214–230. Lea & Febiger, Philadelphia, PA.

Dorland's Illustrated Medical Dictionary, 26th Ed. 1995

Allen, K.G.D. & Klevay, I.M. (1994) Copper: an antioxidant nutrient for cardiovascular health. *Curr. Opinion Lipidol.* 5: 22–28

Lei, K.Y. & Carr, T.P. (eds.) (1990) *Role of Copper in Lipid Metabolism*, p. 179, 201, 217, 233. CRC Press, Boca Raton, FL

O'Dell, B.L. (1990) Copper. In: Present Knowledge of Nutrition (Brown, M.I., ed.) 6th ed., pp. 261–267. International Life Sciences Institute, Washington, DC.

wastewater. This case involved the biological amplification of selenium by aquatic plants which were important in the diets of affected animals.[178]

An extreme case of selenium poisoning

The *Journal of the American Medical Association* recently reported the case of a 36-year old man who was taking 10 vitamin tablets a day containing selenium as an element in holistic therapy for fatigue. During the first week, he developed diarrhea and a tingling sensation in his scalp and extremities. His fatigue worsened and he experienced hair loss. By the end of the second week, he was completely bald. He discontinued the medication, but color changes in his fingernails and toenails developed a few days later, representing heavy-metal poisoning.

High Potency

- High potency vitamins are the trademark of drugs and vitamins, but are not designed by nature. Low potency does not mean foods and whole food concentrate supplements are less effective than synthetic supplements.

- The Daily Value (DV) suggested for vitamins and minerals does not consider the need for micronutrients and quality of nutrients.

[178.] Burk, R.F., ed. (1994) *Selenium in Biology and Human Health*. Springer-Verlag, New York, NY

Combs, G.F., Jr. (1994) Essentiality and toxicity of selenium: a critique of the Recommended Dietary Allowances and the Reference Dose. In: *Risk Assessment of Essential Elements* (Mertz, C., Abernathy, C. & Olin, S.S., eds.), pp. 167–183. International Life Sciences Institute Press, Washington, DC.

APPENDIX C

QUESTIONS & ANSWERS
ON WHOLE FOOD NUTRITION

Vitamins & Drugs Work, Don't They?

QUESTION: With all of the scientific evidence about the wonders of specific vitamins and how they eliminate symptoms and cure disease, how can anyone say that **vitamins do not work**?

ANSWER: There is no doubt that isolated and synthetic vitamins work on symptoms. In fact, drugs also work. And surgery can remove tumors and diseased tissues and organs. You could even say that a tourniquet stops bleeding or that a wad of chewing gum can plug a leaky pipe. But do any of these things really eradicate the *cause* of the problem? Do they heal the wound? Of course not. The main argument posed by a naturalist approach to health care is that vitamins and drugs do not work *in the same way* that natural, whole foods do. Drugs and vitamin pills cause side effects because they both act as pharmacological agents—chemicals that force the body into causing a reaction, generally to stimulate or suppress a biochemical or physiological cellular function. Even so-called "natural" vitamins may create problems in the body because vitamins are singular substances that need many other substances to make them work.

Therefore, when taking a vitamin supplement, the body is forced to surrender various nutrients and chemicals to make the vitamin viable, or to help it work. This takes its toll on the body, creating side effects. Most of the side effects resulting from taking vitamins go unnoticed in the short term, but often create health problems in the long term.

The human body must have real, natural, raw foods to live in a state of health, healing and prevention. Vitamin pills do not provide any nutrients other than isolated vitamins. As human organisms, we absolutely must have a wide array of nutrients (found in the whole food complex) to survive. These nutrients include not only vitamins and minerals, but also trace minerals, enzymes, coenzymes, antioxidants, covitamins, bioflavonoids and more. If these do not come from our diets, then they must come in some sort of supplemental form, such as whole food concentrates.

Foods work nutritionally, while drugs and isolated vitamins work pharmacologically. The former feeds cells recognizable, friendly biochemicals, while the latter only serve to suppress or stimulate bodily functions. The human body knows how to use and easily get rid of food substances, but drugs and vitamins place a burden on the body. We may say that vitamins and drugs work to force the body to accomplish some goal in the same way that pushing a car will move the car when it runs out of fuel.

Studies on Food Nutrients & Their Role in Prevention & Disease

QUESTION: Are there any **studies** that prove that food really makes us healthy?

ANSWER: A few of the many studies proving the health benefits of Nature's foods are included in this book; some appear in this brief section. Other studies are reported regularly in both mainstream and specialized media.

All too frequently people—professionals as well as lay people—flippantly declare there is no proof that foods cure disease or have anything to do with our ability to fight illness. Further, they claim that the use of natural foods to promote health is a matter of pseudoscience and "new age" quackery. This is false. There have been countless studies reported in leading medical and research publications (*Journal of the American Medical Association, Lancet, Journal of Clinical Nutrition,* etc.) that prove certain foods eradicate and prevent disease. This book cites many such studies, from research on the beneficial effects of strawberries to the Norwegian study showing that the intake of foods with vitamin A activity was associated with lower incidence of lung cancer independently of cigarette smoking. A few of examples of food studies follow:

Vitamin A Foods

Example Study #1: This particular Norwegian study (mentioned above, showing that the intake of foods with vitamin A activity was associated with lower incidence of lung cancer independently of cigarette smoking) showed that the same result was extended to women as well as men in the 11-year follow up of the study and in hospital-based case-comparison studies in the United States and in England. There is plenty of scientific evidence, published in scientific journals in the United States as well as the rest of the world, to show the benefits of Nature's foods as healing and preventive agents.

Vitamin C Levels & Disease

Example Study #2: A study from Cambridge University in England shows that people with the highest blood levels of vitamin C are least likely to die from any disease and have the lowest incidence of heart attacks.[179] However, this study does not show that taking vitamin C pills helps to prevent death and heart disease because most of the people in the study were

---

[179.] Lancet, Volume 357, 2001

not taking vitamin pills. It is more likely to show that blood levels of vitamin C are a measure of how many fruits and vegetables a person eats each day and that there is a direct relationship between eating fruits and vegetables and prevention of disease. Each increase in blood level of vitamin C was associated with a related drop in death rate and heart attack. You can decrease your risk for death in general, and heart attacks in particular, just by adding a few servings the right kinds of fruits and vegetables per day.

Vitamin E Foods & Menopause

Example Study #3: A study in the May 2 *New England Journal of Medicine* finds that postmenopausal women who received the most vitamin E from foods—about 10 IU a day—were about 60 percent less likely to die of heart disease than those whose intake of the vitamin was lowest (about 5 IU). Supplements appeared to have no effect. Even without a definitive answer, it still makes sense to get at least the RDA (30 IU) of vitamin E from food. Good sources include seeds and nuts, vegetable oils, wheat germ, tuna fish, and oatmeal.[180]

Vitamin D in Mushrooms

Example Study #4: Regarding vitamin D, the American Society for Clinical Nutrition stated "ergocalciferol [vitamin D] was well absorbed from lyophilized and homogenized wild mushrooms in humans. In addition, the results indicated that the bioavailability of vitamin D from dietary sources can be conveniently studied in humans with such an experimental protocol. In conclusion, mushrooms can be reliably recommended as a natural vitamin D source."[181]

---

180. HealthNews from the publishers of the *New England Journal of Medicine;* OnHealth, 2000 OnHealth Network Company, June 4, 1996

181. American Journal of Clinical Nutrition, Vol. 69, No. 1, 95–98, January 1999; American Society for Clinical Nutrition 1999

Oats & Lower Cholesterol

Example Study #5: "Adding oats to a cholesterol-lowering diet improves the effects of that diet in postmenopausal women with elevated cholesterol levels, according to a study recently published in the *Journal of the American Dietetic Association*. One hundred twenty-seven postmenopausal women (average age of 66 years) with high cholesterol took part in the study. Participants followed the Step I Diet, a cholesterol-lowering regimen recommended by the National Cholesterol Education Program (NCEP), for three weeks. They then added one of four dietary treatments for an additional six weeks: oats/milk, oats/soy, wheat/milk, or wheat/soy. The oats-containing regimens significantly enhanced the cholesterol-lowering effects of the Step I diet, whereas the others did not.[182]

Kidney Stones & Dietary Calcium

Example Study #6: Researcher Rosemary C. Fisher reports, "There have been many studies on the role of nutrition in helping to reduce kidney stones. A recent study conducted at Brigham and Women's Hospital and Harvard Medical School found that previous recommendations to limit dairy products in an effort to reduce the risk of kidney stones was misguided. This study conducted on more than 90,000 women, showed 'that women with the highest intake of dietary calcium had the lowest risk of kidney stones.' Researchers have theorized that this is happening because "calcium is believed to neutralize the absorption of oxalate, a substance that is present in foods such as spinach and beets which has been linked to kidney stone formation. It is very important to note that the reduced risk of kidney stones was not found for those who took calcium supplements. For those taking calcium supplements the risk of kidney stones increased slightly. Researchers theorized that this happens 'because supplements are

---

[182.] Appleton, ND, Jeremy, "Oats Lower Cholesterol In Postmenopausal Women," *Healthnotes Newswire* (December 20, 2001)

often not taken in conjunction with meals, limiting the calcium's ability to neutralize the absorption of oxalate.'"[183]

Apples & Asthma

Example Study #7: "People who eat more apples are less likely to develop asthma than are those who eat few, according to new research published in the *American Journal of Respiratory and Critical Care Medicine*. The study also found that high intake of foods rich in the mineral selenium reduce asthma risk. Among those who already have asthma, consumption of 1 to 2 glasses of red wine per day was associated with reduced severity of the disease. This is the first study to report a protective effect of high apple intake on asthma, and the first to report a protective effect of high red wine intake on asthma severity. Previous research has consistently found reduced levels of selenium in the blood of adults with asthma, so the protective effects of a selenium-rich diet were somewhat anticipated."[184]

Summing Up The Studies

The above studies are just a sampling of the efficacy of real, whole, natural foods on health. Of course there are also innumerable reports filed by the "alternative" health industry, but many of these are anecdotal and lack scientific evaluation because they do not employ the scientific method. This is not to say that anecdotal and historical claims to the effects of foods and herbs are not valid or that they do not suggest the healthfulness of certain foods and herbs, but only that they do not stand up to the critical inspection of the scientific community and are therefore not included as "proof" in this book.

---

183. Fisher, Rosemary C. 1999 [foodandlife.com]

184. Appleton, ND, Jeremy, *Healthnotes Newswire* (December 20, 2001), re: Shaheen SO, Sterne JAC, Thompson RL, et al. Dietary antioxidants and asthma in adults. *Am J Crit Care Med* 2001;164:1823–8

Medical textbooks describe the healing power of foods. In fact, not until it was politically incorrect to do so, modern doctors were telling us that we should get our vitamins and minerals only from our foods. Now that the pharmaceutical industry is leading the way in the vitamin and supplement industry, doctors are no longer standing behind food nutrients as being valuable. To say that there is no scientific proof or medical studies to support food nutrients and their role in health and healing is to speak in total ignorance.

To challenge the healing powers of Nature's foods shows how backwards our thinking has become. Instead of relying on the innate intelligence of Nature and her foods for sustenance, people now generally think that eating is connected only with giving our bodies energy to move through the day. As a modern society, we have lost touch with the healing properties of Nature's foods. Instead, we have been brainwashed into entertaining the ridiculous notion that drugs and vitamins are what's right for our bodies. In fact, many people would rather defend the use of artificial and altered substances than to stand behind what is biologically appropriate for our health. Instead of embracing Nature, modern man, with modern science leading the way, tends to thwart and abuse Nature. We have become accustomed to being impressed by scientific innovation, from space travel to mobile phones, and from gas guzzling, polluting automobiles to foods in bright packages that end up in our trash dumps. We seem especially impressed by the actions of chemicals on our bodies and their ability to mask symptoms and decrease pain.

QUESTION: Drugs and vitamins may be dangerous for our health, but can't the same thing be said about foods in some cases?

ANSWER: The most important way to answer this is to keep the conversation in context. When taken **as intended**, vitamins and drugs create side effects. When taken in excessive dosages, these substances are even more dangerous to human health. Foods, when ingested in their natural states, are known to be edible and nutritious and rarely cause harm. Even when there are problems digesting *good foods*, the severity of sickness rarely approaches the degree that is COMMON with drugs and isolated vitamins, minerals and amino acids.

There are many species of poisonous plants ranging from mushrooms to poison ivy, but these are not considered foods and are not meant to be ingested under any circumstances. Of course there are some foods that may stimulate an allergic reaction in some individuals, but these problems are miniscule in comparison to the widespread health threat posed by isolated chemicals. Some of the allergic reactions to foods are often due more to the treatment of such foods than the foods themselves. For instance, people are not meant to tolerate synthetic fertilizer and pesticide residues on foods and therefore get sick. Many of the side effects or allergic reactions to fruit are owing to sprayed produce, wherein organic produce does not cause the same problems. Further, many allergies to natural foods are due to a faulty or impaired immune system or even deficiencies which, once balanced, result in complete tolerance for the once-offensive foods.

One of the biggest problems these days is that people generally do not understand what their bodies are meant to ingest; and they have not been taught to differentiate between a bag of potato chips and a baked potato in terms of healthfulness. People also tend to overdose on everything, from nonfoods to drugs, and from exercise to the use of herbs. Part of the reason for this is the "more is better" syndrome that we entertain as part of our grandiose way of looking at life, leisure and the pursuit of happiness.

Measuring the Value of Nutrients

QUESTION: How many **milligrams of a vitamin** are in a specific food or whole food concentrate supplement?

ANSWER: The notion of appraising the worth of foods by the quantity of milligrams of their vitamins is an arbitrary rating system that is both misleading and narrow in scope, making people forget about the true value of food in the overall health picture. The milligram and high dosage paradigm is the product of marketing and science, not Nature.

Each and every food is imbued with different quantities of nutrients. No two oranges or carrots are the same, nor do they contain the same amount of vitamin C or carotenoids. Instead of appraising foods for maximum dosages of vitamins and minerals, the naturalist philosophy is to appraise foods for their qualities, completeness and complexities. Micro amounts of vitamins and minerals, when balanced inside whole foods, provide health benefits where megadoses of vitamins fail. When regarding whole food nutrients, we are appreciating the whole food complex rather than arbitrary amounts of individual chemicals. Along the same line of thinking, in some cases a food's chlorophyll content may be the key ingredient to improving your health. Or it may be the bioflavonoids that your body needs even more than the vitamin C. Foods are too complex to judge according to the pharmaceutical paradigm.

Toxicity of Vitamins and Minerals

QUESTION: Are **vitamins toxic?**

ANSWER: Some vitamins are toxic in certain dosages, especially vitamin A, vitamin D and vitamin E. Other vitamins, including niacin, can cause severe health disturbances. Because these substances are not natural, they are always potentially harmful, considering the fact that people self-prescribe, self-medicate and do not understand the dangers inherent in vitamin pills. Liver damage is the most notable toxic side effect of vitamin pills. Other side effects may not be immediately observed.

QUESTION: Are **minerals** safe to take in supplement form?

ANSWER: This always depends upon the individual. However, the truth about minerals is that, as with other nutrients, they exist in a balanced state to achieve and promote optimum health. This is Nature's design. Isolated minerals that are not in food form can easily create a biochemical chain reaction inside our bodies. Unless we know exactly how much of a certain mineral we need to create balance, we run the risk of this chain reaction. For example, if we take zinc we can decrease copper levels; zinc also competes with iron; iron can upset calcium levels; too much magnesium can decrease our use of calcium; fluoride can disrupt thyroid activity and use up calcium supplies; etc. Certain isolated minerals, such as potassium and iron pose a threat to health that has resulted in hospitalization on many occasions.

Excess iron can cause other metals such as copper, calcium and manganese to accumulate in the body by binding with them, and they become deposited in the wrong places and cause harm. Copper is notorious in this respect, especially if the liver is compromised. Manganese can also accumulate in the liver and brain. Calcium can build up in the arteries. Many women with breast cancer have calcium deposits in their breasts and, according to some doctors, only chelation can remove them.[185] Copper tends to antagonize other minerals like zinc, manganese, vitamin B6 and molybdenum.

The late psychiatrist, Dr. Carl Pfeiffer of Princeton University, reported that 64% of his female patients and 37% of males had elevated copper.[186] Women tend to have higher copper levels than men because of their higher estrogen levels. Dr. Pfeiffer correlated high copper levels with high blood pressure, hair loss, PMS, insomnia, tinnitus, depression, schizophrenia, learning disability, autism and hyperactivity.

Excess copper could be in your drinking water or it could be caused by your plumbing. Well water often has high copper levels. In May 1997, about 20 tons of copper was dumped into Lake Ontario. Such dumping began in the 1970s and continued into the 1980s. Smoking, clothing dyes

---

185. *Anticancer Research, 1994*

186. Journal of Orthomolecular Medicine in 1987

(especially dark ones), copper pots, the new high copper amalgam fillings, and herbicides and pesticides can increase your copper levels.

The key concern is how we know exactly how much of any mineral we have circulating or stored in our bodies at any given time. Plus, to manually balance mineral levels we must be able to calculate each mineral's potential interaction with every other mineral. Of course this is impossible, making mineral supplementation a risky business.

Supplements for Athletics

QUESTION: What is the **best regimen for athletes?** Isn't supplementation with amino acids a good idea, as practiced by so many athletes?

ANSWER: Generally speaking athletes who are in highly competitive fields such as bodybuilding, track and field, football, etc. are more interested in improving their game than achieving health. General health concerns and wear and tear on the body are sacrificed for competitive goals. In other words, these people want to eat and take supplements to increase their musculature, endurance, speed, athleticism and strength and mask symptoms rather than to become healthier individuals. This is why they take so many supplements, and why many take a variety of drugs that includes steroids, pain killers, growth hormones and speed. Until an athlete makes health his top priority, he will not be satisfied with whole foods, whole food concentrates or natural health care unless this can be incorporated into a regimen of drugs and artificial stimulants.

Athletes need a variety of food nutrients to provide support to a body under stress and catabolism (breakdown). Foods that provide cellular energy, musculoskeletal repair and support, cardiovascular strength and adrenal backup are highest on the priority list. Complex carbohydrates, pure water, clean air, fruits, eggs and other protein foods, bone meal, yeast, raw nuts and seeds, and plenty of dark green vegetables are highest on the list. Many athletes create a daily health shake "smoothie" that includes a raw organic egg, a banana, strawberries, orange and apple juice blended together with specific whole food concentrates to provide complete proteins, amino acids, carbohydrates, fiber, essential fatty acids, bioflavonoids, antioxidants, chlorophyll, enzymes and more.

Regarding fortifying one's regimen with amino acids, we must admit this, like mineral supplementation, is also risky. Amino acid supplementation has been discussed in detail earlier in this book, but to recap, perhaps it is best to refer to the published works by the late Carl Braverman, M.D. In his book, The *Healing Nutrients Within: Facts, Findings & New Research on Amino Acids,* Braverman demonstrates that amino acids exist in a delicate balance within the human biochemistry, writing:

> The vast field of amino acid interactions is just beginning to unfold. Because many of the amino acids are absorbed and metabolized in a similar fashion, there is a great deal of competition between molecules. sometimes, one amino acid can cancel the effect of others. This adds to the overall complexity of prescribing amino acids to treat disease. For example, amino acids compete for absorption with others in the same group, e.g., the aromatic amino acid group (tryptophan, tyrosine and phenylalanine) and can inhibit one another's passage into the brain. This competition usually occurs among amino acids with similar structure...Amino acids in each group participate in the same or similar actions and perform the same or similar functions, while dissimilar amino acids are absorbed differently and perform different functions.
>
> For example, [the amino acids] taurine and glycine have the same function and compete for absorption. Glutamic acid and aspartic acid have the same function and compete for absorption, but have a function opposite that of [the amino acids] taurine and glycine]....Some amino acids have these kinds of relationships with drugs formed from amino acids that are structurally related to them. An example of this is the amino acid

tyrosine, the metabolism of which is inhibited by the tranquil-izer Haldol (haloperidol) and by the antihypertensive {high blood pressure medication] methyl dopa.[187]

This small excerpt from Braverman's book is enough to show that amino acids represent a highly complex and dynamic subject matter. Not only is there competition between amino acids, but also imbalances resulting from drug use; and there is a constant change in amino acid usage and depletion due to daily diet, exercise, disease, stress and environmental exposure. Toxicity from amino acid supplementation, Braverman points out, is easy to accidentally achieve at doses as low as 50 times the thera-peutic dose range; this may be far less depending on the individual.

On supplementation, Braverman writes:

> The question of supplementing amino acids raises the same problem that once arose with the B vitamins. Early in the use of B vitamin supplements, physicians thought that they all had to be given together. We discovered that multi-B vitamins are not always a good idea. For example, thiamine [vitamin B1] can raise blood pressure; pantothenic acid [vitamin B5] can cause joint pain; too much folic acid can't be tolerated by epileptics or allergy patients.
>
> The same is true for amino acid therapy. Biochemical individu-ality demands the selective use of amino acid supplements for each patient. Different individuals have different amino acid needs; even the amino acid structure of common proteins within differ-ent individuals is different. Multi-amino acid formulas are rarely useful except in patients with generalized amino acid deficiencies (cancer patients, alopecia, anorexia and glucagonoma).[188]

---

187. Braverman, pages 14–15

188. ibid, pages 21–22.

Many amateur athletes and aspiring athletes look with awe upon professional athletes who are extremely muscular in terms of size, and are unnaturally strong. Although most extremely muscular athletes may deny it, the truth is that almost all are involved in taking steroids to achieve their superhuman proportions and strength. The fact that this drug usage is hidden from the public tends to perpetuate the lie that such results may be achieved solely through extreme exercise and diet. Body builders who compete in large tournaments are prime examples of people who use steroids to achieve their muscularity. Getting them to admit their steroid use is next to impossible due to a mixture of egoism and legality.

Most professional athletes take supplements like amino acid shakes and other concoctions containing a host of isolated, synthetic vitamins, minerals, coenzymes and high potency herbs. These are not natural and they are not foods; they may promote strength, endurance, speed and muscular bulk, but they are not health-promoting in any natural sense.

Aren't We Healthier Today?

QUESTION: Aren't **modern peoples healthier today** than ever before in history? Isn't this substantiated by an increased rate of longevity?

ANSWER: We tend to confuse longevity with quality of life. Our nation is overcrowded with nursing homes full of elderly patients who are kept alive only through artificial means. And the population of America is statistically sick, with estimates that show at least 50% of our population is chronically ill, suffering from one sort of illness or another, ranging from recurring headaches and obesity, to backaches and heart disease.

A recent PBS (Public Broadcasting System) documentary reported,"A chronic illness is a condition that lasts a year or longer, limits activity, and may require ongoing care. More than 125 million Americans have at least one chronic condition, such as diabetes, cancer, glaucoma, and heart disease. Nearly half as many have more than one chronic condition…By the year 2020, the number of people living with chronic conditions is expected to rise to 157 million. Direct medical costs associated with these conditions are expected to double to more than $1 trillion—80 percent of the nation's health care spending—while a quarter of the American population is expected to be living with multiple chronic conditions."[189]

And these are only the *reported* conditions!

The rate of cancer continues to escalate, with some studies showing that 50% of all men will end up with cancer, and 33% of all women. Another PBS report shows, "For most people, cancer is a word that generates fear and a great sense of dread, especially for those who have been diagnosed with the disease or know someone who has. And with good cause. This year over a half a million Americans are expected to die from cancer."[190]

More than 600,000 hysterectomies are performed every year. Sherrill Sellman, author of *Hormone Heresy*, says, "One out of three women will have had a surgical menopause before sixty years of age—a hysterectomy that includes removal of the ovaries. To date about 20 million American women have had their uteruses removed. In Europe, the proportion is only one seventh, perhaps because medicine is socialised in several European countries and there is less of a profit motive."[191]

Drug use is out of control, both recreationally and legally (prescription medications). Boasting the highest crime rate in the world, America is emotionally ill as well. Just like our drugs mask our symptoms, our medical approach to illness masks the fact that we are sicker than we seem.

---

189. pbs.org, "Who Cares: Chronic Illness In America,"2001, Fred Friendly

190. pbs.org, "Cancer Warrior," 2001, Rick Groleau and Lexi Krock

191. Sherill Sellman, 2002, home.iae.nl/users/lightnet/health/hysterectom

Look around you and talk to people and you will see that almost everyone has an illness they are dealing with; and everyone knows someone who is dying or has died of cancer or heart disease! Despite the runaway use of vaccines and the empty promises associated with their efficacy, disease rates are climbing.

The most modern nations have all but conquered disease caused by improper sanitation such as poor sewage treatment and disposal and impure indoor air quality, as compared to the late 1800s when such environmental assaults were claiming greater numbers of lives. Much of our uncleanness has in the past contributed to massive disease rates and epidemics. In America, few people live in tents and squalor with dirt floors as witnessed in third world nations. This is more a testimony to our wealth as a nation than it is to health improvements. Now, however, our disease is far more hidden—not only are our symptoms quelled and masked with drugs, but even more startling is the fact that our illnesses are too often the direct result of man's careless and ubiquitous use of chemicals that cause cancer and other diseases. Disease due to industry are back, and causing far more damage to health than ever before. Our environment is toxic and this is affecting all of us, though our corporations will not admit their wrongdoing and we will not hear about environmental disease through our corporate-owned media. Deadly and crippling are the effects of nuclear waste, chemical dumping, chemical spills, air pollution due to factory and automobile emissions, and massive use of pesticides and artificial fertilizers. Fluoride and chlorine, both known by our top scientists as deadly chemicals (industrial waste products), are put into our water systems due to politics, not medical proof. Now our radioactive waste is finding its way into furniture, crops and beef products, being put to use as substances to irradiate germs. This is an evilly clever way for industry to get rid of its cancerous nuclear waste, and the public is being sold a proverbial bill of goods that this waste is beneficial.

As we grow sick from such poisons in our environment, we are being lied to by the corporations that are responsible, as they are telling us through our medical institutions and media, that sickness comes from germs and genetics. This is merely a smoke screen to cover up their irresponsibility, but it is making us sick nonetheless. The diseases of our modern society are not fewer in number; they have merely changed shape. Instead of dying in droves from consumption, people are dying from exposure to man-made chemicals that cause cancer.

Organically Grown Foods

QUESTION: Is there really much of a difference between **organically grown foods** and other produce?

ANSWER: Would you spray a bunch of fresh grapes with a can of Raid bug spray right before you eat it? How about if you rinsed them with a little water first and then put them in your mouth? No? But this is exactly how you eat your fruits and vegetables when they are not organically grown. You may not see the bug spray being applied, but you can be certain it's there just the same. This is only one example of poisoning from the environment that takes its toll on our health. Pesticides are so overused that they show up in all sorts of foods, not just produce. Author John Steinman's *Safe Shoppers Bible* tells us that a typical (non-organic) chocolate chip cookie may contain more than 50 different types of pesticide residues. This is not only a remarkable statement with regard to quantities of pesticides, but more importantly, it reflects how pesticides permeate all non-organic foods, despite whether we are talking about fruits and vegetables or processed foods. Pesticides that are even considered too dangerous for use in the United States are used in other countries; then, ironically, the sprayed foods are imported back here where they show up in our grocery food stores. Pesticides can and do cause cancer, not to mention many other diseases and symptoms from skin eruptions to respiratory ailments.

There is also a nutritive difference between non-organic foods and their organically grown counterparts. Some tests indicate up to 600% more nutrients showing up in organic foods due to better soils, more natural farming conditions and the absence of nutrient damaging pesticides and synthetic fertilizers.

Usually, people buy organic foods for what they DON'T get: pesticide residues, drug and hormone residues (in animal products), and other contaminants such as aluminum, mercury and lead. However, they should also seek organic products for what they DO get: more nutrients and better taste.

A study comparing organically-grown fruits and vegetables to standard ["conventionally grown"] supermarket produce discovered that the organic products averaged 250% more nutrients, with some items containing 500% to 600% more nutrients!

Another study found that organic carrots were brighter in color, firmer and stronger (better) tasting than conventional carrots. A French study revealed that organically-grown carrots contained more beta-carotene (and other carotenes) and organic celeriac contained more vitamin C complex than their conventionally raised counterparts.

Modern, mechanized, mass-production farming methods using chemical fertilizers and increasingly more toxic pesticides on produce and grains, as well as growth hormones, antibiotics, sulfa drugs, and other medications administered to animals in addition to their pesticide-laden feed, results in foods that are of poor quality, lack flavor, contain lower values of nutrients, and have poisonous residues. Such food is raised to look good, not to provide high nutritional quality or to be safe.

Few persons under the age of 50 know what really good food tastes like unless they are eating organically. When an elderly person complains that foods just don't taste like they used to, this is not necessarily a consequence of aging. Foods grown organically taste better because they contain the nutrients derived from rich soil as nature intended. Additionally, they are not a source of toxic substances. Pesticides alone have been shown to cause neurological problems, birth defects, and cancer, for example.[192]

The subject of pesticides and their potential health risks is vast enough for an entire book and years of study. Pesticides are created to kill; they are chemicals of mass destruction. While political speeches made by presidents and military leaders focus on the threat of annihilation at the hands of armies and weapons, this even greater menace is largely ignored even though it is not just a threat, but rather an ongoing, escalating reality responsible for killing and destroying human lives in our country every moment of every day. There is a rising sentiment that promoters and producers of life-threatening fake foods and harmful chemicals are engaged in the most un-American of all activities even as they hide behind our laws to conduct their unethical business practices. The enemy is within.

Common sense alone dictates that we are all better off eating natural, organically grown foods to avoid eating cancer-and disease-causing chemicals, despite how loud big industry is screaming that their chemicals are safe and effective.

---

192. DeCava, Judith A., "Are You Eating Poisoned Foods? Organically Grown Foods Offer More than Just Safer Nutrition...," *Health X Files Newsletter*, Creative Bureau Publishing, 1997

APPENDIX D

RESOURCES

WHOLE FOOD CONCENTRATE SUPPLEMENTS

NutriPlex Formulas, Inc.
P.O. Box 17482
Boulder, CO 80301
www.nutriplexformulas.com

Nutrition Research Center
www.nutritionresearchcenter.org

GREAT BOOKS

Illness Isn't Caused by a Drug Deficiency!
Vic Shayne, Ph.D.

Whole Food Nutrition: The Missing Link in Vitamin Therapy
Vic Shayne, Ph.D.

Toxic Sludge is Good For You!
Sheldon Rampton & John Stauber

Trust Us, We're Experts!
Sheldon Rampton & John Stauber

Chinese System of Food Cures
Dr. Henry C. Lu

Food: Your Miracle Medicine
Jean Carper

Staying Healthy With the Seasons
Elson Haas, M.D.

Diet for a New America
John Robbins

Vibrant Health From Your Kitchen
Dr. Bernard Jensen

Empty Harvest
Dr. Bernard Jensen

Food & Healing
AnneMarie Colbin

The Green Pharmacy
James Duke, Ph.D.

Inventing the AIDS Virus
Peter Duesberg, Ph.D.

Food Is Your Best Medicine
Henry Bieler, M.D.

RECOMMENDED WEBSITES

prwatch.org
wri.org
projectcensored.org

devc.org
nutritionresearchcenter.org
freespeech.org
savewhatsleft.org
greenpeace.org
enn.com
scorecard.org

0-595-23654-5

www.ingramcontent.com/pod-product-compliance
Lightning Source LLC
Chambersburg PA
CBHW061351280526
45784CB00001B/219